IMMUNOLOGY

An Illustrated Outline

Second edition

IMMUNOLOGY

An Illustrated Outline

Second edition

DAVID MALE MA PhD

Senior Lecturer in Neuroimmunology
Institute of Psychiatry
London SE5

Gower Medical Publishing · London · New York

Distributed in the USA and Canada by:
J B Lippincott Company
East Washington Square
Philadelphia
PA 19105
USA

Distributed in the UK and Continental
Europe by:
Gower Medical Publishing
Middlesex House
34-42 Cleveland Street
London W1P 5FB
UK

Distributed in Australia and New Zealand
by:
Harper and Row (Australia) Pty Ltd
PO Box 226
Artarmon
NSW 2064
Australia

Distributed in Southeast Asia, Hong
Kong, India and Pakistan by:
Harper and Row (Asia) Pte Ltd
37 Jalan Pemimpin 02-01
Singapore 2057

Distributed in Japan by:
Nankodo Co Ltd
42-6 Hongo 3-chome
Bunkyo-ku
Tokyo 113
Japan

Project Manager	**Claire Hooper**
Designer	**Jane Brown**
Illustrators	**Jane Brown**
	Catherine Duffy
Production	**Susan Bishop**
Publisher	**Fiona Foley**

Originated in Hong Kong by Bright Arts.
Setting & Page make-up on Apple Machintosh.
Output by Text Unit, London.
Text set in Univers. Captions in Helvetica narrow.
Produced by Mandarin offset. Printed in Hong Kong.

Library of Congress Cataloging-in-Publication Data
Male, David K. 1954 -
    Immunology: An Illustrated Outline / David Male - 2nd ed.
    p. cm.
    Includes Index
    1. Immunology - Outline, syllabi. etc. 2. Clinical Immunology -
    Outlines, syllabi. etc. I. Title.
    [DNLM: 1. Allergy and Immunology - Outlines. QW518 N245u]
    QR 182.55.M35 1991

British Library Cataloguing-in-Publication Data
    Male, David
    Immunology: An Illustrated Outline. - 2nd ed.
    I. Title
    616.07

ISBN 0-397-44825-2

How to Use This Book

This book serves two different functions. It can be used either as a dictionary of immunology or as a concise revision guide/study aid. Readers who already know some immunology and require a summary of particular aspects, should consult the contents page. The book is divided into six chapters each of which contains a number of related topics.

To use the book as a dictionary, look up the word or abbreviation in the Index of Terms (pages viii to xv). This gives a single page number where a definition of the word will be found-associated words will be found on the same page. Page references to particular topics set out on several pages are indicated in bold figures.

Acknowledgements

I am most grateful to my coeditors Professor Ivan Roitt and Dr Jonathan Brostoff for letting me use or adapt some of the illustrations which previously appeared in our book *Immunology*. I would like to thank the contributors who inspired those diagrams, including Professors Frank Hay and Michael Steward, and Drs Peter Lydyard, Anne Cooke, Graham Rook, Michael Owen, Marc Feldmann, James Howard and Malcolm Turner. In addition, I would also like to thank Dr B. Greenwood, Professor C.H.W. Horne, Dr B. Dean, Professor L. Brent and Dr C. Hawkins for original micrographs and illustrations of pathology.

Naturally a book of this kind cannot include everything of interest to immunologists; I have tried to cover all the essential areas of the subject, but I should be pleased to know when the readers consider that particular subjects deserve further detail.

Contents

4. Inflammation and Cell migration

5. Immunopathology

6. Immunological Tests and Techniques

INDEX OF TERMS

The Immune System   1

INTRODUCTION

The function of the immune system is to protect the body from
damage caused by invading microorganisms – bacteria, viruses,
fungi and parasites. This defensive function is performed by leucocytes (white blood cells) and a number of accessory cells,
which are distributed throughout the body, but are found particularly in lymphoid organs, including the bone marrow, thymus
spleen and lymph nodes. Large accumulations of these cells are
also found at sites where pathogens may enter the body, such
as the mucosa of the gut and lung. Cells migrate between these
tissues via the blood stream and lymphatic system. As they do
so, they interact with each other to generate coordinated
immune responses aimed at eliminating pathogens or minimiz-
ing the damage they cause.

Lymphocytes are the key cells controlling the immune
response. They specifically recognize 'foreign' material and distinguish it from the body's own components. Generally they
react to foreign material but not against the body's tissue.
Lymphocytes are of two main types: B cells which produce antibodies, and T cells which have a number of functions including:
1) helping B cells to make antibody; 2) recognizing and destroying cells infected with viruses; 3) activating phagocytes to
destroy pathogens they have taken up; and 4) controlling the
level and quality of the immune response. Lymphocytes recognize foreign material by specific cell-surface antigen receptor
molecules. To specifically recognize the enormous variety of
different molecules, the antigen receptors must be equally
diverse. Each lymphocyte makes only one type of antigen
receptor, and thus can only recognize a very limited number of
antigens. But since the receptors differ on each clone of cells,
the lymphocyte population as a whole has a great diversity of
specific antigen receptors.

Phagocytes include blood monocytes, macrophages and neutrophils. Their function is to take up pathogens, antigens and
cell debris and to break it down. Antibodies and complement components bound to particles facilitate this process,
and macrophages can also present internalized antigens to lymphocytes.

Accessory cells include eosinophil and basophil granulocytes, mast cells, platelets and antigen-presenting cells (APCs). Eosinophils have a role in damaging some parasites and controlling inflammation. Basophils, mast cells and platelets contain a variety of molecules that mediate inflammation, and so are important in linking immune responses to inflammatory reactions. Antigen-presenting cells include several cell types which present antigen to lymphocytes. All these cell types interact to generate an effective immune response.

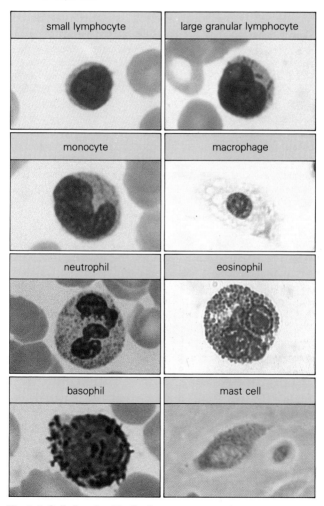

small lymphocyte	large granular lymphocyte
monocyte	macrophage
neutrophil	eosinophil
basophil	mast cell

Fig. 1.1 Cells involved in the immune response.

LYMPHOCYTES

B Cells are lymphocytes which develop in foetal liver and subsequently in bone marrow. In birds B cells develop in a specialized organ, the bursa of Fabricius. Mature B cells carry surface immunoglobulin which acts as their antigen receptor. They are distributed throughout the secondary lymphoid tissues, particularly in the follicles of lymph nodes and spleen. They respond to antigenic stimuli by dividing and differentiating into plasma cells, under the control of cytokines released by T cells.

Plasma cells/Antibody Forming Cells (AFCs) are terminally differentiated B cells. They have an expanded cytoplasm with characteristic parallel arrays of rough endoplasmic reticulum and are entirely devoted to the production of secreted antibody. Plasma cells are seen in the red pulp of the spleen, the medulla of lymph nodes, the MALT and in small numbers at sites of inflammation.

B cell subsets. In man, the majority of B cells are derived from bone marrow stem cells, but a minor population, distinguished by the CD5 marker, appear to form a self renewing set. Cells within this set develop early, respond to a number of common microbial antigens and sometimes generate autoantibodies. In mice, a subset of B cells expressing Lyb5 distinguishes cells which can respond to a particular group of T-independent antigens.

T cells are lymphocytes which develop in the thymus. This organ is seeded by lymphocytic stem cells from the bone marrow during embryonic development. These cells then develop their T cell antigen receptors (TCRs) and differentiate into the two major peripheral T cell subsets, one of which expresses the CD4 marker and the other CD8. T cells can also be differentiated into two populations depending on whether they use an α/β or a γ/δ type of antigen receptor. The essential role of T cells is to recognize antigens originating from within cells of the host. Different populations of T cells have different functions, as follows:

T helper (T$_H$) cells. These T lymphocytes help B cells to divide, differentiate and produce antibody. They also release cytokines which control the development of leucocyte lines from haemopoietic stem cells. Other cytokines are required for the development of cytotoxic T cells and cause activation of macrophages, allowing them to destroy the pathogens they have taken up. The majority of T$_H$ cells are CD4$^+$ and recognize antigen presented on the surface of antigen-presenting cells in association with class II molecules encoded by the major histocompatibility complex (MHC).

3

TH1/TH2 cells are subsets of T helper cells differentiated *in vitro* according to the blends of cytokines they produce. TH1 cells may promote delayed hypersensitivity reactions while TH2 cells release cytokines which are particularly required for B cell differentiation. Both types can promote development of cytotoxic cells.

T delayed hypersensitivity (TD) cells are the T cells responsible for bringing macrophages and other inflammatory cells to areas where delayed hypersensitivity reactions occur. These appear to be a particular functional group of TH cells.

T cytotoxic (Tc) cells are capable of destroying virally-infected target cells, or allogeneic cells. The majority of Tc cells are CD8+ and recognize antigen on the target cell surface associated with MHC class I molecules

T suppressor (Ts) cells are functionally defined T cells which downregulate the actions of other T cells and B cells. Although many studies have identified CD8+ Ts cells, there is no unique marker for this group of cells, and it is suspected that suppression may be a facet of the regulatory actions of TH and Tc cells.

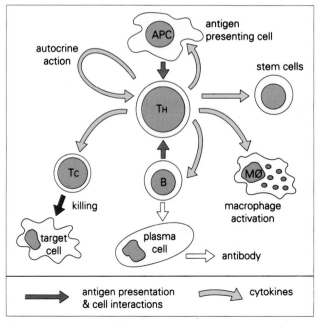

Fig. 1.2 Interactions of T helper cells.

Clonal selection describes the way in which particular lympho-cytes are activated. During development each lymphocyte gener-ates an antigen receptor with a single antigen specificity, but the entire population of cells has a very wide range of specificities. An antigen binds specifically to only a few cells. These clones alone are stimulated to divide, so providing a large pool of effector cells and memory cells. Thus antigen selects specific clones.

Memory cells are populations of long-lived T cells or B cells which have been previously stimulated by antigen, and make an acceler-ated response to that antigen if they encounter it again. Memory B cells carry surface IgG as their antigen receptor, and this is of higher affinity than on virgin lymphocytes. Memory T cells may be distinguishable by high expression of CD44.

Virgin lymphocytes are cells which have not encountered their specific antigen.

Null (Non-T, non-B) cells/L cells/Third population cells are all descriptions of a distinct population of leucocytes constituting 14% of blood mononuclear cells. They lack conventional antigen receptors, but express some markers from both the T cell and mononuclear phagocyte lineages. Nevertheless, they are thought to constitute a distinct lineage. These cells have a high density of Fc receptors (FcγRIII) which permits them to recog-nize and kill target cells coated with antibody. Seventy to eighty per cent of these cells have the appearance of large granular lymphocytes.

Large Granular Lymphocytes (LGL) is a morphological descrip-tion of a population of lymphocyte-like cells containing large amounts of cytoplasm with azurophilic granules. They constitute 5–15% of blood mononuclear cells, and seem to correspond with mature null cells. This population has particular K cell and NK cell activity.

K (Killer) cells are mononuclear cells that can kill target cells sensi-tized with antibody, which they engage via their Fc receptors. The majority are null cells, although macrophages or eosinophils can also have K cell activity.

NK (Natural Killer) cells are capable of killing a variety of virally-infected and transformed target cells to which they have not been previously sensitized. Their receptor for the target cells is not clearly defined, but is not a conventional antigen receptor molecule. Most have LGL morphology.

Effector and Target cells are functional descriptions applied where any cell type (effector) acts upon another (target), but particularly where the effector kills the target.

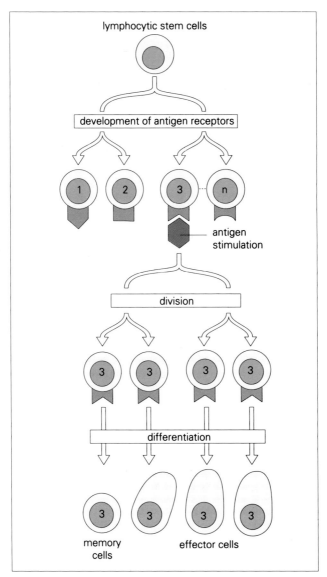

lymphocytic stem cells

development of antigen receptors

1 2 3 n

antigen stimulation

division

3 3 3 3

differentiation

3 3 3 3

memory cells

effector cells

Fig. 1.3 Clonal selection.

MARKERS

Lymphocytes and other leucocytes are differentiated by their cell surface molecules identified by monoclonal antibodies. The most readily accessible marker of lymphocytes is their antigen receptor – B cells use surface immunoglobulin and T cells carry the T cell antigen receptor (TCR). Other markers are designated according to the CD system of nomenclature. Some of these markers are specific for individual populations of cells, or particular phases of cellular differentiation. Others appear only on activated or dividing cells. However, many of the CD markers are present at varying levels on several different cell types. Nevertheless, each subset of lymphocytes expresses a unique overall profile of surface markers.

CD markers. This system of nomenclature is used for leucocyte surface molecules, as identified by monoclonal antibodies. More than 80 individual molecules are recognized by this series, and some of them are found on cells other than leucocytes. The table opposite gives the identity and cellular distribution of the more important CD molecules. The most frequently encountered CD molecules are those used to distinguish T cells: CD2 is present on all T cells and is involved in antigen-non-specific activation; CD3 is present on all T cells. It is an invariant part of the T cell antigen receptor and is involved in antigen-specific T cell activation; CD4 occurs on TH cells and is involved in MHC class II restricted interactions; CD8 occurs on Tc cells and is involved in MHC class I restricted interactions.

Thy-1 (θ), an allelically variable molecule encoded on mouse chromosome 9, is present on all T cells but also occurs in brain.

Ly (Lyt) antigens. These are a large series of cell surface molecules found on mouse T cells. Ly1 (CD5) identifies the major helper cell population in this species, whereas Ly2,3 (CD8) distinguishes Tc cells.

L3T4 is the mouse equivalent of CD4.

Lyb antigens are surface markers of mouse B cells. The Lyb5 antigen identifies a subset of B cells which is responsive to a particular group of T independent antigens.

α**-Naphthyl acid esterase (ANAE)** is an enzyme which appears as a few clustered dots on stained T cells and also occurs diffusely in mononuclear phagocytes.

Acid phosphatase is seen in T cells, but also occurs in neutrophils, eosinophils and null cells.

	M_r kD	identity/function	T cell	B cell	null cell	monocyte/ macrophage	granulocyte
CD1	45	differentiation marker	Thy				
CD2	50	antigen-non-specific activation					
CD3	16-26	TCR-subunit					
CD4	59	MHC class II receptor					
CD5	67	differentiation marker					
CD8	32	MHC class I receptor					
CD11a	180	LFA-1 (α chain)					
CD11b	155	CR3 (α chain)					
CD11c	150	CR4 (α chain)					
CD16	50-65	FcRIII					
CD18	95	β_2-integrin chain (see CDII)					
CD19	95	differentiation marker					
CD20	32-37	differentation marker					
CD21	140	CR2					
CD23	45-50	FcεRII				*	Eo
CD25	55	IL-2 receptor (β chain)	*	*		*	
CD29	130	β_1-integrin chain (see CD49)					
CD32	40	FcRII					
CD35	160-250	CR1					
CD44	80-95	Pgp-1 adhesion molecule					
CD45	200	leucocyte common antigen (LCA)					
CD45R	~200	restricted LCA					
CD46	56-66	membrane cofactor protein (MCP)					
CD49a	210	VLA-1 (α chain)	*				
CD49b	167	VLA-2 (α chain)	*				
CD49d	150	VLA-4 (α chain)					
CD54	76-114	ICAM-1	*	*	*		
CD55	70	decay accelerating factor (DAF)					
CD56	135/220	NKH1	*	*			
CD57	110	HNK1					
CD58	40-65	LFA-3					
CD64	75	FcRI					
CD71	95	transferrin receptor	*	*	*	*	

present   subset only   * activated cells   useful marker

Eo = Eosinophil   Thy = Thymocytes

Fig. 1.4 CD markers.

ANTIGEN-PRESENTING CELLS

Antigen Presenting Cells (APCs) are a group of functionally defined cells which are capable of taking up antigens and presenting them to lymphocytes in a form they can recognize. Some antigens are taken up by APCs in the periphery and transported to the secondary lymphoid tissues, while other APCs are normally resident in these tissues and intercept antigen as it arrives. Whereas B cells recognize antigen in its native form, TH cells recognize antigenic peptides which have become associated with MHC molecules. Consequently, in order to present antigen to a TH cell, an APC must internalize it, process it into fragments, and re-express it at the cell surface in association with class II MHC molecules. In addition, many APCs provide additional stimuatory signals to lymphocytes either by direct cellular interactions or by cytokines. The characteristics of the main APCs of spleen and lymph node are shown below.

Langerhans' cells (veiled cells) are recirculating cells found in skin which pick up antigen and transport it to regional lymph nodes. They express CD1 and high levels of MHC class II

APC	Region	MHC Class II	Present to
marginal zone macrophage	spleen lymph node	–	B cells
macrophage	circulatory lymphoid tissue	– → +	B&T cells
Langerhans' cell veiled cell dendritic cell	skin afferent lymph lymph node (paracortex)	++ ++ ++	virgin T cells
dendritic leucocyte	tissues	++	T cells
follicular dendritic cell	lymphoid follicles	–	B cells
B cell	lymphoid tissue	+ → ++	T cells

Fig. 1.5 Antigen Presenting Cells.

molecules and have a characteristic racket-shaped granule, the Birbeck granule (function unknown). In afferent lymph they are seen as veiled cells, and in lymph nodes as dendritic cells. They are particularly important in the development of contact hypersensitivity, and skin-sensitizing agents induce their emigration from skin.

Dendritic (Interdigitating) Cells (IDCs), located in the T cell areas of lymph nodes, express class II MHC molecules and are very effective in presenting antigen to virgin CD4$^+$ T cells.

Dendritic leucocytes are resident cells distributed throughout most of the tissues of the body, and are thought to be related to the dendritic cells of lymphoid tissues.

Follicular Dendritic Cells (FDCs) are present in spleen and lymph node follicles, where they appear tightly surrounded by lymphocytes. Complement-fixing immune complexes localize on the surface of these cells via Fc and C3 receptors, where they are presented mainly to B cells. This form of complex localization and presentation is important in the development of B cell memory.

Marginal zone macrophages are present in the marginal zone of the splenic PALS and along the marginal sinus of lymph nodes. T-independent antigens such as polysaccharides tend to localize on these cells, where they are often very persistent. They present antigens primarily to B cells.

Antigen-presenting macrophages. Macrophages phagocytose antigens and some of them can also process and present it. The recirculating macrophages of secondary lymphoid tissues are mostly seen in the medulla of lymph nodes and the red pulp of spleen. They are particularly effective in presenting antigens to T cells which have been previously sensitized.

Facultative antigen presenting cells. Many cells of the body can be induced to express MHC class II when stimulated by IFN-γ from activated T cells. Sometimes they are able to present antigen to CD4$^+$ T cells, although they are often only weakly active, presumably due to their inability to deliver costimulatory signals. Antigen presentation by such cells may even render them more susceptible to killing by cytotoxic cells.

Nurse cells are thymic epithelial cells seen *in vitro*. They are closely surrounded by developing thymocytes. Antigen presentation by these cells is important in the development of the T cell repertoire.

PHAGOCYTES AND AUXILIARY CELLS

Mononuclear phagocyte system (MPS)/reticuloendothelial system is the collective term for the long-lived phagocytic cells distributed throughout the organs of the body. They are derived from bone marrow stem cells and express receptors for immunoglobulin (FcRI) and complement (CR1, CR3 and often CR4). They phagocytose antigenic particles and some have the ability to present antigen to lymphocytes. This group includes:

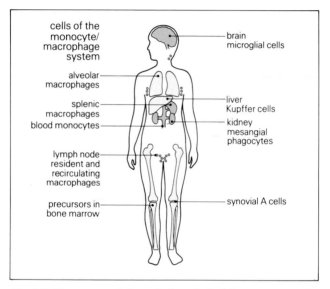

Fig. 1.6 Phagocytes of the reticuloendothelial system.

Monocytes circulating cells, constituting about 5% of total blood leucocytes, which can migrate into tissues to become macrophages. These cells have a horse-shoe shaped nucleus, azurophilic granules and many lysosomes.

Macrophages are large phagocytic cells found in most tissues and lining serous cavities and the lung. Resident macrophages may remain in tissues for years whereas others recirculate through secondary lymphoid tissues, where they may function as APCs.

Kupffer cells are phagocytes which lie along the liver sinusoids. Much of the antigen entering the body through the gut is removed by these cells.

Mesangial phagocytes line the glomerular endothelium where the capillaries enter the Bowman's capsule.

Microglial cells are resident phagocytes of brain which they enter around the time of birth.

Synovial A cells are one of the cell types which lie on the synovium, in contact with the synovial fluid.

Granulocytes (polymorphs), recognizable by their multilobed nucleii and numerous cytoplamic granules, constitute the majority of blood leucocytes. They are classified according to their histological staining as:

Neutrophils are professional phagocytes and the most abundant of the leucocytes (>70%). They spend less than 48 hours in the circulation before migrating into the tissues under the influence of chemotactic stimuli, where they phagocytose material and eventually die. They have receptors for antibody and complement to facilitate uptake of opsonized particles.

Eosinophils comprise 2 – 5% of blood leucocytes. Their granules contain a crystalloid core of basic protein which can be released by exocytosis causing damage to a number of pathogens, particularly parasites. The granules also contain histaminase and aryl sulphatase which down-regulate inflammatory reactions.

Basophils constitute <0.5% of blood leucocytes. Their granules contain inflammatory mediators and they are in some ways functionally similar to mast cells.

Mast cells are present in most tissues adjoining the blood vessels. They contain numerous granules with inflammatory mediators such as histamine and PAF, released by triggering with C3a and C5a, or by crosslinking of surface IgE bound to their high affinity IgE receptor (FcεRI). Stimulation also causes them to produce prostaglandins and leukotrienes. There are two types of mast cell:

Connective Tissue Mast Cells (CTMC) are the main tissue fixed mast cell population. They are ubiquitous, contain large amounts of histamine and heparin and unlike MMCs are susceptible to the action of sodium cromoglycate.

Mucosal Mast Cells (MMCs) are present in the gut and lung. They are dependent on T cells for their proliferation and are increased during parasitic infections.

12

LYMPHOID SYSTEM

Primary and Secondary lymphoid tissue. Lymphocytes are developed from bone marrow stem cells, and initially develop in the primary lymphoid tissues – T cells in the thymus and B cells in bone marrow. Mature cells expressing antigen receptors seed the secondary lymphoid tissues, the spleen, lymph nodes and collections of mucosa-associated lymphoid tissues (MALT).

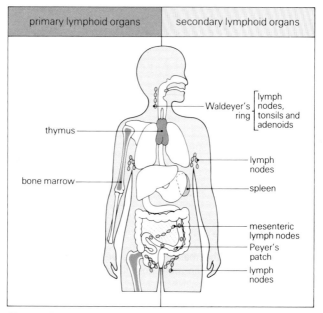

Fig. 1.7 Major lymphoid organs and tissues.

Lymphocyte traffic/recirculating cells. Lymphocytes leave the circulation by traversing specialized venules (HEV) in the lymph nodes and MALT. These cells recirculate via the lymphatic system through chains of lymph nodes back to the circulation. Macrophages and Langerhans' cells also recirculate from the periphery to lymph nodes where they can present antigen to the lymphocytes.

High endothelial venules (HEV) are present in most secondary lymphoid tissues, and may be induced in other tissues during severe, persistent immune reactions. They are lined by distinctive columnar cells, expressing specific adhesion molecules. A high proportion of lymphocytes passing through secondary lymphoid tissues bind to these molecules and migrate across this endothelium.

Lymphatic system is the system of vessels covering the entire body, which is responsible for draining tissues and returning the transudate to the blood. It also acts as a channel for the movement of antigens from the periphery to lymph nodes, and for the recirculation of lymphocytes and macrophages.

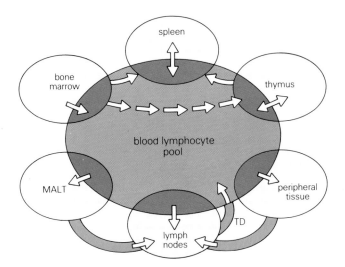

Fig. 1.8 Lymphocyte traffic.

Thoracic duct is the main lymphatic vessel through which recirculating cells pass en route from the trunk, internal organs and lower limbs, to the circulation. It drains into the left subclavian vein.

Right lymphatic duct drains the upper right segment of the body.

Mucosa-Associated Lymphoid Tissue (MALT) is a general term for the unencapsulated lymphoid tissues, which are seen in submucosal areas of the respiratory, gastrointestinal and urinogenitary systems. These protect sites of potential pathogen invasion.

Tonsil, a pharyngeal part of the MALT, is particularly rich in B cells and is arranged into follicles.

Waldeyer's ring is the term for the lymphoid tissue of the neck and pharynx, which includes the adenoids, tonsils and regional lymph nodes.

LYMPH NODES

Lymph nodes are encapsulated organs which punctuate the lymphoid network, and contain aggregations of lymphocytes and antigen presenting cells. They are strategically placed to intercept antigens from the periphery and there are large groups of lymph nodes in the axillae, groin and neck. The mesenteric lymph nodes are very large, and well sited to protect the body from antigen and pathogens from the gut. Lymph nodes are structurally organized into different areas:

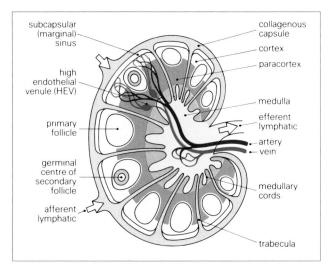

Fig. 1.9 The structure of a lymph node.

Marginal sinus lies immediately beneath the capsule and is lined by phagocytic cells, the marginal zone macrophages, which can trap antigens entering the node.

Cortex, the outer region of the lymph node, contains mainly B cells. Follicles lie within this region.

Lymphoid follicles are aggregations of closely packed lymphocytes and APCs. Unstimulated lymph nodes contain primary follicles, which develop into expanded secondary follicles after antigen stimulation.

Germinal centres are regions of rapidly proliferating cells seen in the centre of some secondary lymphoid follicles. The centres contain large and small follicle centre cells (centroblasts and centrocytes), a few CD4$^+$ T cells and follicular dendritic cells, which are important in the development of B cell memory. Around this is the mantle zone, an area of densely packed cells.

Paracortex contains mainly T cells, interspersed with interdigitating cells expressing high levels of MHC class II antigens, which present antigen to the T cells.

Medulla contains relatively fewer lymphocytes and more macrophages and plasma cells than other regions.

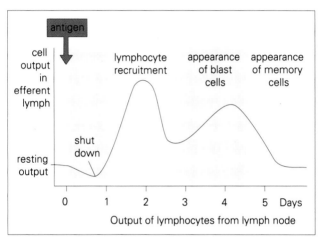

Fig. 1.10 Output of lymphocytes from lymph nodes.

Medullary cords are strands of lymphocytes, both B and T cells, which extend into the medulla.

Afferent and Efferent lymphatics. Cells arrive in the lymph nodes via the HEV and afferent lymphatics which drain into the marginal (subcapsular) sinus. From here they migrate across the node, or into specialized areas, and finally leave by the efferent lymphatic vessel.

Lymph node shutdown. Under normal circumstances there is a steady efflux of lymphocytes from a lymph node, but when antigen enters the node of a sensitized animal, the emigration stops for a period of about 24 hours, referred to as shutdown. This is followed by an enhanced outflow as lymphocytes are recruited to the node. After a few days antigen-specific lymphocytes begin to emerge. 16

SPLEEN

The spleen is an encapsulated secondary lymphoid organ which lies in the peritoneum, beneath the diaphragm and behind the stomach. It contains two main types of tissue, termed the red pulp and the white pulp or PALS.

Red pulp consists of a network of splenic cords and venous sinuses lined by macrophages, which effect the destruction of effete erythrocytes. Plasma cells may also be seen in this region.

White pulp/PALS (Periarteriolar Lymphatic Sheath) contains the majority of the lymphoid tissue, distributed around the arterioles. T cells are found mainly around the central arterioles and B cells further out. The B cells may be organized into primary and secondary lymphoid follicles, with germinal centres. Phagocytes and APCs are also present in the follicles.

Marginal zone is the outer region of the PALS. It contains slowly recirculating B cells and marginal zone macrophages which present T-independent antigens to B cells. Marginal sinuses lie at the edge of the marginal zone. Most lymphocytes enter the PALS via specialized capillaries in the marginal zone and migrate out via bridging channels, between the marginal sinuses, into the venous sinuses of the red pulp.

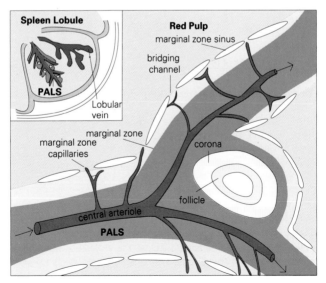

17   **Fig. 1.11 The Periarteriolar Lymphatic Sheath (PALS).**

GALT (GUT ASSOCIATED LYMPHOID TISSUES)

The GALT is the mucosa-associated lymphoid tissues of the gut. This includes the focal accumulations of lymphocytes in the lamina propria and Peyer's patches, which contain disproportionately high numbers of IgA producing B cells and plasma cells.

Peyer's patches are collections of lymphocytes in the wall of the small intestine, which appear macroscopically as pale patches on the gut wall. The adjoining part of the intestinal mucosa lacks goblet cells and has a specialized epithelium that includes a unique cell type, the M cell, which transports antigens to the underlying lymphocytes. Here also, IgA produced locally is transported to the gut lumen. Lymphocytes enter a patch via the HEV, which expresses organ-specific adhesion molecules, before distributing to the B and T cell areas.

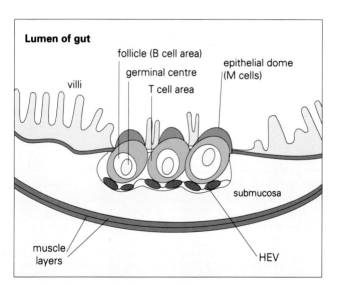

Fig. 1.12 Structure of Peyer's patch.

Secretory immune system refers to immune defences present in secretory organs, such as salivary glands, mammary glands and GALT. The main protection is provided by secretory IgA. Dimeric IgA binds to a poly-Ig receptor on the basal surface of epithelial cells and is transported to the gut lumen.

THYMUS

The thymus is a primary lymphoid organ overlying the heart, seeded by lymphoid stem cells from the bone marrow, which differentiate into T cells. It is bilobed and organized into lobules separated by connective tissue septae (trabeculae). Each lobule is divided into cortex and medulla.

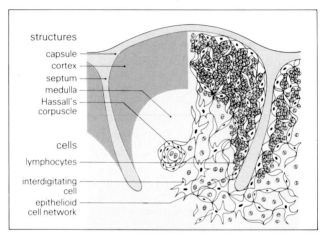

Fig. 1.13 The structure of a thymus lobule.

Thymocytes are thymic lymphocytes. The repertoire of T cell antigen receptors develops and the deletion of autoreactive cells occurs, during T cell maturation in the thymus, by interaction with APCs. The process involves proliferation of immature cells, but many cells die (by apoptosis) during selection.

Thymic cortex. The outer zone contains about 85% of the total thymocytes. The cells are immature, express CD1 in man and divide rapidly.

Thymic medulla contains relatively few lymphocytes but they are more mature than those in the cortex and the peripheral T cell populations (CD4+ or CD8+) start to emerge here.

Thymic epithelial cells are a network of MHC class II bearing APCs extending throughout the cortex and medulla, which are thought to be involved in the selection of the T cell repertoire.

Hassal's corpuscles are whorled structures, possibly of epithelial cells, seen in the medulla. Their function is unknown.

LYMPHOCYTE DEVELOPMENT

Bone marrow is a haemopoietic tissue present in some bones. A network of venous sinuses is arranged around a central artery and vein and these permeate the developing cells. All blood cells are derived from bone marrow stem cells and 10% of marrow cells are lymphocytes, occurring in clusters around the radial arteries. In adult mammals, B cells develop and differentiate here.

Education of T cells occurs in the thymus, following seeding by pre-T cells from bone marrow. The most immature cortical thymocytes are CD4$^-$,8$^-$ but these develop into the rapidly proliferating CD4$^+$,8$^+$ population, which constitutes the majority of thymocytes. These cells subsequently generate their antigen receptors (TCR), and undergo positive and negative selection. The differentiating thymocytes lose either the CD4 or the CD8 marker to leave mature T cells expressing only CD4 or CD8, which are seen in the medulla.

Positive and Negative selection. The process by which T cells which can respond to antigen in association with their own MHC molecules are selectively expanded while self-MHC reactive cells are deleted during thymic development. The process is thought to involve interaction with thymic cortical epithelium and thymic APCs respectively.

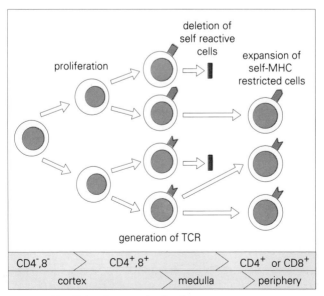

Fig 1.14 T cell development in the thymus.   20

Immune Recognition | **2**

ANTIGEN RECEPTORS

The immune system has two main ways of recognizing antigens. B cells recognize intact antigens using immunoglobulin (antibody) as their receptor. T cells on the other hand have evolved to recognize antigen originating from within other cells using their T cell antigen receptors (TCR).

Antigen is the term used to describe any molecule that can be recognized by the immune system. In general, immunoglobulins recognize and bind to intact antigens, or large fragments of them which have retained their tertiary structure. By contrast, T cells will only recognize polypeptide fragments of antigens which have become associated with molecules encoded by the major histocompatibility complex (MHC) and which are expressed on the surface of other cells of the body.

Antigenic determinant or epitope is the part of an antigen to which an immunoglobulin binds. Antigens usually have many determinants which may be different from each other, or be repeated molecular structures. Virtually the entire surface of a protein is potentially antigenic. Figure 2.1 illustrates the epitopes on lysozyme.

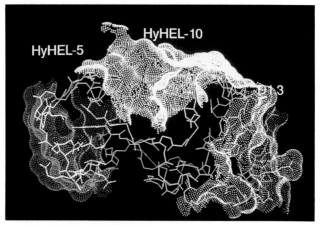

Fig. 2.1 Epitopes of lysozyme. Courtesy of Dr D.R. Davis.

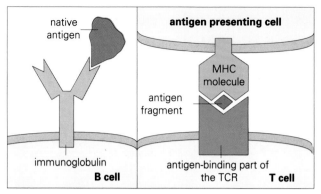

Fig. 2.2 Antigen receptor molecules.

Antibodies (Abs)/Immunoglobulins (Igs) were originally identified as a class of serum proteins induced following contact with antigen, which bind specifically to the antigen that induced their formation. Most antibodies are present in the gamma globulin fraction of serum. Subsequently it was found that B cells use a membrane bound form of their secreted antibody as an antigen receptor.

T cell antigen receptors (TCR) are integral membrane proteins on all mature T cells, which specifically recognize antigenic peptides associated with MHC-encoded molecules. The receptor consists of a heterodimer responsible for antigen/MHC binding and a cluster of associated membrane bound polypeptides which trigger cellular activation. The term Ti is used to describe the antigen/MHC binding portion of the TCR, which varies between different clones of T cells. The associated polypeptides of the TCR do not vary between T cells and are often referred to as the CD3 complex. CD3 is a marker of mature T cells.

MHC class I and II molecules present antigen to T cells. They do this by combining with polypeptide fragments of antigens within cells, which are then transported to the cell surface. Class I molecules are present on all nucleated cells of the body, but class II molecules only on a restricted group of antigen-presenting cells.

Associate recognition describes the way in which the TCR recognizes a unique combination of a particular antigenic peptide associated with an MHC molecule of a specific haplotype. The TCR interacts with both the peptide and with amino acid residues around the antigen-binding pocket on the MHC class I or class II molecule.

ANTIBODY STRUCTURE

Heavy chains and light chains. Antibody molecules all have a basic four polypeptide chain structure, consisting of two identical light (L) chains and two identical heavy (H) chains, stabilized and crosslinked by intra-chain and inter-chain disulphide bonds (red), and the heavy chains are glycosylated (blue). There are five major types of immunoglobulin heavy chains (μ, γ, α, ϵ, δ) consisting of 450 - 600 amino acid residues and the type determines the class of the antibody. Light chains are of two main types (κ, λ) consisting of about 230 residues, and either type of light chain may associate with any of the heavy chains. Both heavy and light chains are folded into domains.

Membrane and Secreted immunoglobulins. Antibodies can either be produced as integral membrane proteins of B cells, which act as their antigen receptor, or in a secreted form. Secreted immunoglobulins are structurally identical to their membrane counterparts except that they lack the transmembrane segment and small intracytoplasmic section of amino acids at the C-terminus of membrane Ig. Secreted Igs are present in extracellular fluids and secretions. Virgin B cells produce membrane immunoglobulins, but following activation by antigen and differentiation into plasma cells, they switch to the production of secreted Igs.

Domains are globular regions of proteins. Antibody domains consist of 3 or 4 polypeptide loops stabilized by β-pleated sheet and an

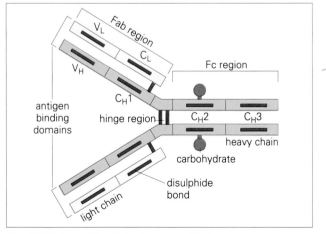

Fig. 2.3 Polypeptide chain structure of IgG.

intra-chain disulphide bond. The structure so formed is sometimes called a β-barrel. Light chains have two domains and heavy chains four or five.

The hinge region is a section of the heavy chain between the Fc and Fab regions which contains the inter-heavy chain disulphide bonds and confers segmental flexibility on the antibody molecule.

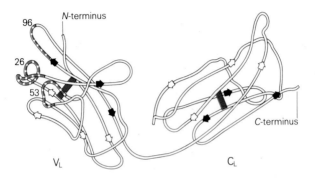

Fig. 2.4 The basic folding pattern of the variable and constant domains of the light chain.

Variable (V) and Constant (C) regions. Examination of the degree of amino acid variability between different antibody molecules of the same class shows that the largest amount of sequence variation is concentrated in the N-terminal domains of the light and heavy chain; hence this is called the V region. The V regions of one light and one heavy chain form an antigen binding site. The remaining domains are relatively invariant, within any particular class of antibody and so are called the constant (C) region. The domains of antibody molecules are named according to whether they are in the variable or constant region of the molecules, and according to whether they are in the light or heavy chain. For example:

V_H and V_L are the variable domains of heavy and light chains.

C_L and C_H1 are the constant domains of the light chain and the first constant domain of the heavy chain, respectively.

$C\gamma$, $C\mu$, etc. Heavy chain domains are sometimes referred to by the class of antibody. For example $C\mu1$ is the first constant domain of the μ heavy chain of IgM antibody.

ANTIBODY - STRUCTURAL VARIATIONS

Antibody molecules are structurally heterogeneous even though they are all built up from units which have the basic four polypeptide chain structure.

Classes and subclasses. Antibodies may be grouped on the basis of structural similarities into different classes and subclasses depending on their heavy chains. Each class subserves different functions. In mammals there are five antibody classes – IgG, IgM, IgA, IgD and IgE. IgG and IgA are further divided into subclasses. The number of subclasses varies between species. For example, in man there are four IgG subclasses, IgG1 – IgG4. The subclasses are isotypic variants.

Kappa and Lambda chains. Antibody light chains may also be divided into two types namely κ and λ which are encoded by separate gene loci. Both types of light chain can combine with any of the heavy chains.

Allelic exclusion is the process by which a cell uses either the gene from its maternal chromosome or the one from the paternal chromosome, but not both. Individual B cells display allelic exclusion of their heavy and light chain genes.

The variability of antibodies is due to their being encoded by a number of genes which are rearranged before they are expressed. Variation may be divided into three categories:

Isotypes are variants which are present in all members of a species, for example the different antibody classes and subclasses where there are distinct genes for each variant lying within the immunoglobulin heavy chain gene cluster.

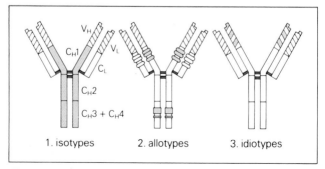

1. isotypes   2. allotypes   3. idiotypes

Fig 2.5 Variability of immunoglobulin structure.

Allotypes are variants due to intraspecies genetic differences. Each individual has a particular variant at each Ig gene locus, which will often differ from those in other individuals.

Idiotypes are variants due to the large amount of structural heterogeneity in the immunoglobulin V regions, related to the great variety of V domains required to bind diverse antigens.

Kabat and Wu plot shows the amino acid sequence variability in immunoglobulins, determined by comparing the amino acid sequences of many different antibodies. It plots variability against amino acid position, thereby highlighting the most variable regions of the heavy and light chains.

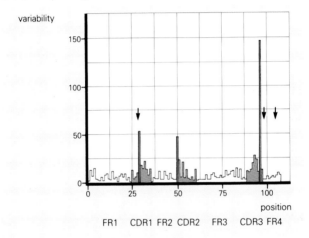

Fig. 2.6 Kabat and Wu plot of light chain variability.

Hypervariable regions and Framework segments Using the Kabat and Wu technique on immunoglobulin V regions it is found that most variability is clustered in three hypervariable regions (red) separated by relatively invariant framework segments (FR).

Complementarity Determining Region (CDR) is virtually synonymous with a hypervariable region and is a part of the V region which forms the antigen binding site. V domain folding brings the CDRs together at the distal tip of the molecule.

Groups and Subgroups The numerous V region domains can be classified into groups and subgroups according to similarities in the amino acid sequences of their frameworks. The genes for members of a particular group are often contiguous.

ANTIBODY FUNCTIONS

Antibodies are bifunctional molecules. Their first function is to bind antigen and the second is to interact with host tissues and effector systems to facilitate removal of the antigen. Some antibody functions can be mediated just by binding to the antigen. For example antibodies which bind to surface molecules of viruses can prevent their binding to and infecting host cells. However most antibody functions require that the complexed antigen is bound to Fc receptors on cells. The antigen-binding sites are formed by the V domains of a heavy and light chain, whereas the C domains of the Fc region interact with cells of the immune system and C1q of the complement system. The different antibody classes and subclasses interact with different cells, and so have slightly different functions.

IgG is the major serum immunoglobulin and constitutes the main antibody in the secondary immune response to most antigens. In man, it is transferred across the placenta to provide protection in neonatal life. All IgG subclasses, except IgG4, can bind to C1q by sites in Cγ2 to activate the complement classical pathway. IgG can act as an opsonin by crosslinking immune complexes to Fc receptors on neutrophils and macrophages. It can also sensitize target cells for destruction by K cells.

IgM is a pentamer of the basic four chain structure. It is the first class to be produced during the development of the immune system and in the primary immune response. It fixes complement very efficiently and is the main antibody component of the response to T-independent antigens.

IgA occurs as monomers, dimers and polymers of the basic four chain unit, existing in man mostly as monomers and in other species as dimers. IgA is the most abundant immunoglobulin class in secretions where it protects mucous membranes. It is also found in colostrum and is particularly important in protecting the neonates of species which do not transfer IgG across the placenta.

J chain is a polypeptide present in polymeric immunoglobulins (IgM and IgA) which facilitates polymerization. It is synthesized by B cells, but is not encoded by the Ig genes.

Poly-Ig receptor is present on the serosal surface of epithelial cells, which can transport and secrete IgA. It is a member of the immunoglobulin supergene family, which has five domains. IgA dimers bind to the receptor and are transported across the endothelium. The receptor is then cleaved, forming the secretory piece and releasing secreted IgA by exocytosis.

Secretory piece is the released form of the poly-Ig receptor, which attaches to IgA by disulphide bonds and is wound around the IgA, to protect it from degradation by enzymes.

IgD is a trace Ig in serum but acts as a cell surface receptor on many B cells, where it is coexpressed with IgM. IgD appears on differentiating B cells following activation, but is absent from mature antibody forming cells.

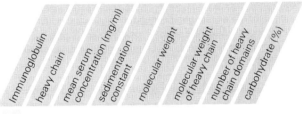

Immunoglobulin	heavy chain	mean serum concentration (mg/ml)	sedimentation constant	molecular weight	molecular weight of heavy chain	number of heavy chain domains	carbohydrate (%)
IgG1	γ_1	9	7S	146,000	51,000	4	2-3
IgG2	γ_2	3	7S	146,000	51,000	4	2-3
IgG3	γ_3	1	7S	170,000	60,000	4	2-3
IgG4	γ_4	0.5	7S	146,000	51,000	4	2-3
IgM	μ	1.5	19S	970,000	65,000	5	12
IgA1	α_1	3.0	7S	160,000	56,000	4	7-11
IgA2	α_2	0.5	7S	160,000	52,000	4	7-11
sIgA	α_1 or α_2	0.05	11S	385,000	52-56,000	4	7-11
IgD	δ	0.03	7S	184,000	69,700	4	9-14
IgE	ε	0.00005	8S	188,000	72,500	5	12

Fig. 2.7 Physicochemical properties of human Ig subclasses.

IgE binds to high affinity Fc receptors (FcεRI) on mast cells and basophils, where it sensitizes them to release pharmacological mediators after contact with antigen. IgE may be particularly important in protection against helminth infections, but it also mediates type I hypersensitivity reactions, such as asthma and hayfever.

ANTIBODY GENES

The genes for antibodies lie at three gene loci on separate chromosomes. These are the κ, λ (L) and heavy (H) chain genes. At each of these loci, there are large numbers of different gene segments, encoding polypeptides (exons), separated by segments which do not encode protein, but which contain sequences important in gene control and the process of recombination (introns). The antibody genes undergo a number of recombinational events during B cell development, and maturation. The first events are DNA rearrangements of H and L chain genes which form the gene segments encoding their V domains. These segment are spliced to the gene segments encoding the C domains to produce mRNA for the H and L chains. At a later stage in development B cells can make further DNA rearrangements associated with switching the class of antibody they produce.

Generation of diversity refers to the process by which the large number of antibody V regions are generated. This is achieved by: 1) a large number of germline V region genes in the separate gene pools for κ, λ and H chains; 2) recombination between V, D and J gene segments; 3) recombinational inaccuracies; 4) somatic point mutations; and 5) the varied combinations of light and heavy chains.

Germline genes are those which are passed down from one generation to the next. They may be altered during cellular development. The main modification of Ig genes is the recombination between V, D and J gene segments which encode the variable domains of the H and L chains, This occurs only in B cells.

V genes encode the N-terminal 95 (approx) amino acids of the antibody V domains. The number of V genes at each locus varies between loci and species, but may be several hundred. Analagous V genes are present at the gene loci encoding T cell receptor (TCR) chains.

J genes and D genes. To produce a gene encoding a H chain V region, any one of the H chain V gene segments is recombined with any of a small number of D (diversity) and J (joining) genes to produce a VDJ gene. Recombination of light chains is similar except that they have no D gene segments, and a V gene is recombined directly to a J gene. Analagous J gene segments are present in the loci encoding the TCR chains and analagous D genes are present in the β and δ loci of the TCR. (Note that J gene segments should not be confused with J chains.)

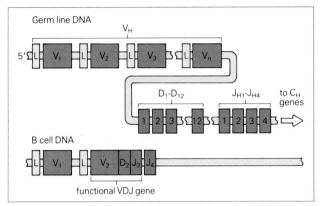

Fig. 2.8 VDJ recombination

Recombination and the 12/23 rule. Recombination is the process by which the various gene segments for antigen receptors are brought together and joined. This process depends on specific recombination sequences flanking each V, D and J gene. The recombination sequences appose the gene segments which are enzymically cut and rejoined to remove the intervening introns. The sequences consist of a heptamer, 12 or 23 bases and a nonamer. The 12/23 rule states that a flanking sequence with 12 bases can only recombine with one of 23 bases. This ensures that heavy chains only make VDJ recombinations and light chains VJ recombinations. The precise point of the recombination may vary, as illustrated below, for the recombination of $V_\kappa 21$ and J_1 in three different myelomas. This gives rise to different base sequences encoding amino acids 95 and 96, thus providing an additional source of diversity.

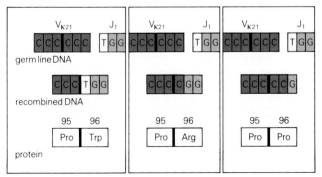

Fig. 2.9 Light chain diversity created by variable recombination.

N regions are sections of nucleotides which become inserted into the junctions between V, D and J gene segments during recombination. They are not encoded in the germline, and are an additional source of diversity.

RAG-1 (Recombination Activating Gene) is thought to control the initiation of recombination in both T cells and B cells.

Somatic hypermutation is the process by which DNA base changes occur during the lifetime of a B cell producing point mutations in the immunoglobulin polypeptides. The rate of mutation is extremely high in the region around the Ig genes. The mechanism becomes activated as B cells differentiate and is associated with, but not consequent on, class-switching. Thus IgG molecules usually vary more from germline sequences than IgM.

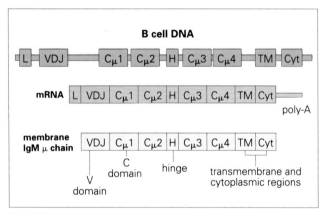

Fig. 2.10 Production of antibody polypeptides.

Antibody synthesis. The segment of DNA encoding the recombined VDJ (heavy chain) or VJ (light chain) region and the C region is transcribed into a primary RNA transcript, which still contains the introns and which can be found in heteronuclear RNA (hnRNA). The primary transcript is then spliced to remove the introns, a process which involves recognition of specific base sequences called donor and acceptor junctions, immediately flanking the exons. This leaves mRNA which is translated across the membrane of the endoplasmic reticulum (ER). Each mRNA has a leader (L) or signal sequence (SS) by which it is directed to the ER. The process is illustrated below for a membrane IgM μ polypeptide. Complete immunoglobulins are assembled and glycosylated within endo-plasmic reticulum, and stored in the Golgi apparatus. Secreted immunoglobulins are released by exocytosis, while membrane Igs are moved to the cell surface.

C genes. The heavy chain constant region genes are arranged downstream (3') of the recombined VDJ gene. Each gene consists of a series of exons encoding the individual C domains as well as separate exon(s) for the hinge (except IgA) and for the transmembrane and cytoplasmic regions. The primary transcript of the heavy chains can be processed in two different ways, to produce mRNA for either membrane or secreted immunoglobulin. To produce membrane immunoglobulin, the exons for the transmembrane segments are spliced to a point just within the final C domain. If this does not occur the stop signal is retained and mRNA for secreted immunoglobulin is produced. The point of polyadenylation controls how the hnRNA will be spliced. Initially a B cell joins a μ gene to its VDJ gene, but other C genes may alternatively be linked to VDJ - this is called class switching.

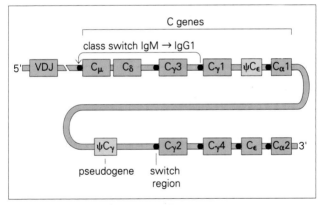

Fig. 2.11 Human Ig H chain gene locus.

Class switching is a process by which the cell can switch the class of immunoglobulin it produces while retaining the same antigen specificity. All the heavy chain constant region genes except δ are preceded by a switching sequence. Switching is effected by bringing a new C gene up to the position occupied by the μ C gene, with the loss of the intervening C genes. This process is illustrated above for the switch from IgM to IgG1. It is also possible for a cell to switch classes by producing very long primary RNA transcripts, which are then spliced to connect the new C gene to VDJ. Indeed this is the only way that IgD (which lacks a switch sequence) can be produced. This process is controlled by T cells and is modulated by cytokines.

ANTIBODY FRAGMENTS

Much of the early work on the elucidation of antibody structure was performed using fragments of antibodies prepared by a combination of methods, including enzyme digestion and selective reduction of the interchain disulphide bonds. The fragments are separated chromatographically. Of particular interest are the Fab and F(ab')2 fragments. Fab has one antigen combining site and so cannot crosslink antigenic determinants, whereas F(ab')2 has two sites and can crosslink antigen. Both lack the Fc region, and are therefore useful in determining which antibody functions are Fc dependent. The table below illustrates the structures of the fragments (yellow) and their means of production. IgG fragments are illustrated, but analagous fragments can be made from other classes of immunoglobulins.

Fragment	Structure	Produced by
F(ab')$_2$	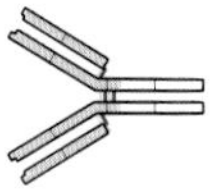	pepsin digestion
Fab'	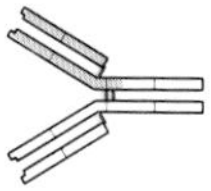	pepsin digestion and partial reduction
Fab	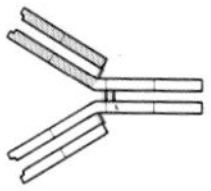	papain digestion
Fc	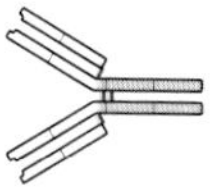	papain digestion
Facb	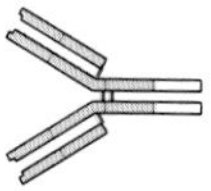	plasmin digestion
pFc'	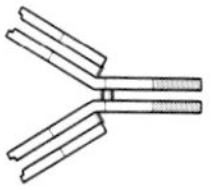	pepsin or plasmin digestion
Fd	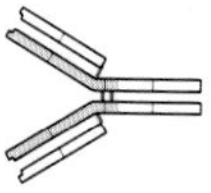	pepsin digestion partial reduction and reaggregation

Fig. 2.12 Antibody fragments.

IDIOTYPES

Idiotopes. Idiotypes (Ids) are variants of immunoglobulins, differentiated according to their different V regions, using anti-idiotypic antibodies. The V domains of different antibodies can act as antigens, just as any other protein can, and antibodies raised to them will recognize different antigenic determinants in the V domains. These are termed idiotopes. An idiotype is effectively defined according to the collection of different idiotopes it expresses.

Cross-reactive idiotypes (CRIs) are analagous to cross-reacting antigens. Sometimes a particular idiotope occurs on two different antibodies, and these will both react with the same anti-idiotypic antibody – i.e. they cross-react.

Idiotype and/or Prototype Ab	Antigen	Strain	Ig Haplotype
TI5	PC	BALB/c	a
NP^b,B(1-8)	NP	C57BL/6	b
ABA(CRI)	ARS	A/J	e
A5A	Streptococcal carbohydrate	A/J	e
MOPC-460	TNP-Levan	BALB/c	a
Dex	α 1,3 Dextran	BALB/c	a
GAL	β 1,6 D-Galactan	BALB/c	a

Fig. 2.13 Examples of mouse idiotypes.

Idi and Idx are abbreviations meaning a unique or individual idiotype (Idi) or a cross-reactive idiotype (Idx). These terms are applied in the context of particular antibody systems.

Recurrent and Dominant idiotypes. Sometimes a particular idiotype is frequently seen in the immune response of different individuals to a particular antigen. This is a recurrent idiotype. If an idiotype constitutes a major part of the antibody response to an antigen then it is a dominant idiotype.

Germline idiotypes. Within inbred groups of animals the ability to produce particular idiotypes often depends on the immunoglobulin haplotype. This is due to the strain having particular sets of antibody V, D and J genes. The table above gives examples of germline idiotypes in mice.

34

ANTIGENS

Immunogens. An antigen is any molecule recognized by the immune system, but the term immunogen is reserved for those antigens which elicit a strong immune response, particularly in the context of protective immunity to pathogenic organisms.

Antigenic determinant is the part of the antigen which binds to antibody (epitope). Antigens usually have many determinants which may differ from each other or be repeated structures.

Haptens and Carriers. Artificial antigens have been used to examine the immune response. In particular small antigenic determinants (haptens) are covalently coupled to larger molecules (carriers). Haptens bind to antibodies but cannot by themselves elicit an antibody response. Haptens are usually recognized by B cells and carriers by T cells.

Carrier Effect. This is the phenomenon where an optimal secondary response is obtained when the hapten is coupled to the same carrier for both the primary and secondary immunization. This is exemplified in Fig 2.15., 1 and 2, in the anti-DNP response following immunization with the carrier-hapten conjugates BSA-DNP and OA-DNP. The carrier effect may be bypassed by priming the animals to the new carrier (OA) before challenge (in Fig 2.15.,3). This is called carrier priming.

ARS	–	Azophenyl arsonate
BGG	–	Bovine gamma globulin
BSA	–	Bovine serum albumin
CGG	–	Chicken gamma globulin
DNP	–	Dinitrophenyl (hapten)
GAT	–	Glutamine Alanine Tyrosine copolymer
KLH	–	Keyhole Limpet Haemocyanin
NIP	–	4-hydroxy, 3-iodo, 5-nitrophenyl acetyl (hapten)
NP	–	4-hydroxy, 5-nitrophenyl acetyl (hapten)
OA	–	Ovalbumin
PC	–	Phosphorylcholine (hapten)
PLL	–	Poly-L-Lysine
(P,G)-A--L;	–	Synthetic polymers with an Ala-Lys (A–L)
(T,G)-A--L;		copolymer backbone substituted with a
(H,G)-A--L;		Glutamic acid (G) and either Phenylalanine (P)
		Tyrosine (T) or Histidine (H) side chains
PPD	–	Purified protein derivative (of tuberculin)
TNP	–	Trinitrophenyl (hapten)
TMA	–	Tetramethyl ammonium (hapten)

Fig. 2.14 Commonly used carriers and haptens.

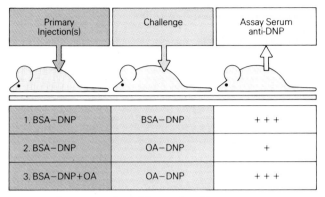

Primary Injection(s)	Challenge	Assay Serum anti-DNP
1. BSA–DNP	BSA–DNP	+ + +
2. BSA–DNP	OA–DNP	+
3. BSA–DNP+OA	OA–DNP	+ + +

Fig. 2.15 Demonstration of the carrier effect.

T-dependent antigens need to be recognized by both T cells and B cells to elicit an antibody response. Most protein antigens fall into this category.

T-independent antigens can stimulate B cells to produce antibody without T cell help. Most are large polymeric molecules with repeated antigen determinants which are only slowly degraded.

Type I and II T-independent antigens are differentiated according to their ability to activate different B cell subsets. Type I antigens stimulate both $Lyb5^+$ and $Lyb5^-$ cells (mouse), whereas type II antigens can only act on $Lyb5^+$ cells.

antigen	polymer	B cell mitogen	resistance to degradation	type
lipopolysaccharide (LPS)	+	+++	+	1
PPD	–	+++	+	1
dextran	++	–	++	2
levon	++	–	++	2
ficoll	+++	–	+++	2
polymerized flagellin	++	+	+	2
poly I: poly C	++	++	+	2
poly D amino acids	+++	–	+++	2

Fig. 2.16 Commonly used T-independent antigens.

ANTIGEN/ANTIBODY INTERACTIONS

Epitopes and Paratopes are part of a nomenclature used to describe the interaction between antigen and antigen receptor molecules, including antibodies. An epitope is an antigenic determinant and the paratope, formed by the hypervariable loops of the V domains, is the part of the antibody which binds to the epitope.

Contact residues are the amino acids of the epitope and paratope which contribute to the antigen/antibody bond.

Continuous and Discontinuous epitopes. Study of the precise molecular interaction between antigen and antibody shows that some epitopes are formed by one linear stretch of amino acids (continuous epitope). In most cases, however, an epitope has contact residues derived from different sections of a protein antigen, brought together by folding of the polypeptide chain (discontinuous epitope).

Antigen/antibody bond. Antibodies bind specifically to the antigen which induces their formation, by multiple non-covalent bonds, including Van der Waal's forces, salt bridges, hydrogen bonds and hydrophobic interactions. Crystallographic studies of immune complexes between antibodies and protein antigens indicates that they interact by complementary surfaces of up to 1000Å^2 with the third hypervariable regions (VJ and VDJ) lying near the centre of the binding site. Hypervariable regions of both L and H chains contribute contact residues. The diagram opposite (top) shows lysozyme antigen (green) and the light (yellow) and heavy (blue) chains of a complexed anti-lysozyme antibody. The lower diagram shows the molecules rotated forward 90° with contact residues (red and pink) numbered on the interacting faces.

Charge neutralization refers to the observation that charged contact residues on an epitope are often neutralized by residues of an opposite charge on the paratope. This is particularly important at the centre of the binding site.

Induced fit refers to the flexing of residues in the hypervariable loops in contact with the epitope which may occur to allow an optimum fit between the interacting molecules.

Antibody affinity is a measure of the bond strength between a single epitope and a paratope. It depends on the sum of the bond energies of the non-covalent interactions, set against the natural repulsion between molecules and the energy required to make any necessary distortions to allow binding (induced fit).

Antibody valency describes the number of binding sites on an molecule. For example IgG has two sites and IgM ten, although the effective number depends on the configuration of the antigen.

Antibody avidity is the total strength of an antigen/antibody bond, which is related to the affinity of the paratope epitope bonds and antibody valency. Binding energy is much enhanced when several bonds form, so avidity usually exceeds affinity.

Cross reaction. Some antisera are not totally specific for their inducing antigen but bind related (cross-reacting) antigens, either due to sharing a common epitope, or because the molecular shapes of the cross-reacting antigens are similar.

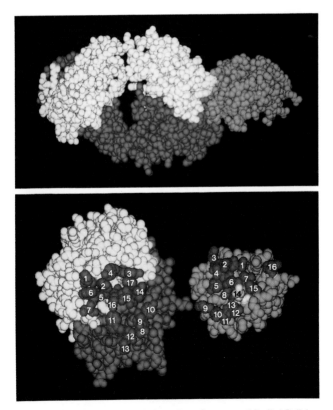

Fig. 2.17 The Fab-lysozyme complex. Courtesy of Dr R.J.Poljak; from *Science* (1986) **233**, 747-753. Copyright 1986 by the AAAS.

T CELL ANTIGEN RECEPTOR (TCR)

The T cell antigen receptor (TCR) consists of a heterodimer (Ti), and a number of associated polypeptides which form the CD3 complex. The dimer recognizes processed antigen associated with an MHC molecule, and the CD3 complex is involved in signal transduction and activation of the T cell.

$TCR_{\alpha\beta}$ (TCR2) and $TCR_{\gamma\delta}$ (TCR1). The polypeptide chains for the antigen-binding portion of the receptor are encoded by four different gene loci α, β, γ and δ, and any one T cell will express either a α/β or a γ/δ receptor. The great majority of thymocytes and peripheral T cells have a $TCR_{\alpha\beta}$, Cells bearing $TCR_{\gamma\delta}$ are a small minority population found in the gut, and to a lesser extent in skin.

Ti is a term used to distinguish the antigen/MHC binding portion (which differs between cells), from the monomorphic CD3 complex. Ti has 4 domains – the N-terminal domains are variable (V) and form the antigen/MHC receptor, whereas the membrane proximal domains are constant (C).

CD3 complex in man consists of four polypeptide chains, each of which span the cell membrane. These are the γ, δ, ϵ and ζ chains. The first three are structurally related, single domain members of the immunoglobulin supergene family, whereas the ζ chains are unrelated and form ζ-ζ dimers. In mouse a fifth chain η is also present, possibly as a minority alternative partner for ζ chains as a $\eta\zeta$ dimer. Following occupancy of the TCR by antigen/MHC, chains of the CD3 complex are phosphorylated, and this is thought to be important in the control of T cell activation.

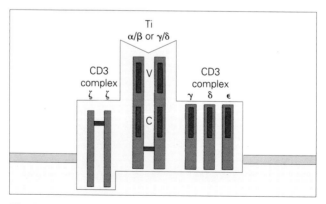

Fig. 2.18 T cell receptor.

T CELL RECEPTOR GENES

The genes for the antigen/MHC binding portion of the TCR are similar to those of antibody, in that they consist of multiple V, D and J segments which become recombined during T cell development to produce functional VDJ or VJ genes (See pages 29 - 32). These encode the N-terminal variable (V) domains of the TCR. The α and γ loci have V and J segments only whereas β and δ have V, D and J segments. The recombined V gene is linked to the exons for the C domains, the short hinge-like section (containing the interchain disulphide bond), the transmembrane and cytoplasmic segments. The layout of the human α and β loci are shown below and that of the mouse α, β and δ loci is very similar. Note that there are tandem sets of genes for the β chain D, J and C regions. Each locus is distinct although the δ chain D, J and C genes lie between the V_{α} and J_{α} genes. The process of recombination can permit variability in the precise linking position of V to J, the possibility of linking the D segments in all 3 reading frames, and the addition of N-region diversity - i.e. bases inserted into the junctions, which are not encoded in the germline. Theoretically the arrangement of recombination sequences flanking the D_{β} and D_{γ} genes permit the assembly of genes with more than one D region (i.e. VDDJ). In contrast to antibody genes, the TCR genes do not undergo somatic hypermutation. Nevertheless the amount of diversity that can be generated is at least as great as for antibodies. The genes for the γ, δ and ϵ polypeptides of the CD3 complex do not undergo any rearrangements and are closely linked on chromosome 11 in man. All CD3 genes are required for TCR expression and charged residues in the CD3 chain transmembrane segments are thought to be involved in association with Ti.

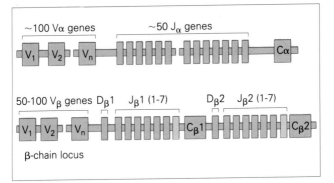

Fig. 2.19 T cell receptor α and β gene loci.

MHC MOLECULES

Major Histocompatibility Complex (MHC) is a large group of genes including those encoding the class I and II MHC molecules, which are involved in presentation of antigen to T cells. The complex was originally identified as a locus encoding allogeneic molecules present on the cell surface involved in graft rejection. It is now known that MHC molecules are essential for recognition of antigen originating within cells.

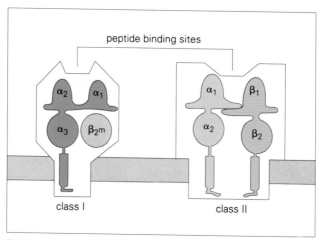

peptide binding sites

α_2 α_1

α_3 β_{2m}

class I

α_1 β_1

α_2 β_2

class II

Fig. 2.20 MHC molecules domain structure.

MHC class I molecules are integral membrane proteins found on all nucleated cells and platelets. These are the classical transplantation antigens. They each have one polypeptide chain encoded within the MHC which traverses the plasma membrane. The extracellular portion has three domains ($\alpha_1 - \alpha_3$). The membrane proximal α_3 domain is associated with β_2-microglobulin, while the two N-terminal domains form an antigen-binding pocket consisting of a base of β-pleated sheet derived from both α_1 and α_2 surrounded by two loops of α-helix. Residues facing into the binding pocket vary between different molecules and haplotypes, to allow different antigenic peptides to bind. The α_3 domain has a binding site for CD8.

β_2-microglobulin is a polypeptide chain encoded by genes outside the MHC, and which forms a single domain, related to Ig domains. It is necessary for transport of class I molecules to the cell surface and their expression there.

MHC class II molecules (Ia antigens) are expressed on B cells macrophages, monocytes, APCs and some T cells. They consist of two non-covalently linked polypeptides (α and β), both encoded by the MHC, which traverse the plasma membrane, each having two extracellular domains. It is thought that class II molecules resemble class I molecules, with the N-terminal α_1 and β_1 domains forming the peptide binding site.

Invariant chains (Ii) are associated with class II molecules during their biosynthesis, but become dissociated as the molecules move to an acidic endosome compartment, where they are thought to associate with antigenic peptides.

MHC class III molecules are a variety of proteins, including various complement components and cytokines.

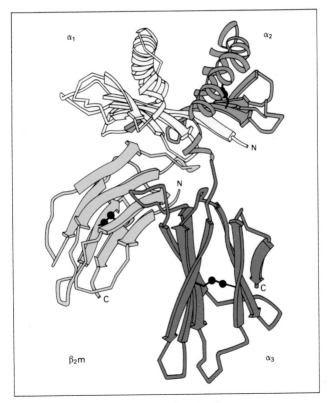

Fig. 2.21 Structure of class I MHC molecule.

42

MHC GENES

H-2 is the mouse major histocompatibility complex which lies on chromosome 17. There are five main regions K, A, E, S and D. Genes with immunological functions in each of these regions are shown below. Pseudogenes have been omitted.

H-2K and H-2D encode class I MHC molecules, the classical transplantation antigens. The K locus has one gene, whereas the number of genes in the D locus varies between strains.

H-2A and H-2E (I-A and I-E) encode the α and β chains of the class II molecules. This was previously designated the H-2I region and subdivided into I-A and I-E.

H-2S contains genes for the complement components C2, factor B (Bf) and C4, as well as the cytokines TNF-α and TNF-β, and a variety of other enzymes.

Slp (sex limited protein) is a non-functional variant of C4.

Qa and Tla loci lie downstream of the H-2 complex and contain genes for more than 25 class IV genes. They may function as haemopoietic differentiation molecules, but may also be a source of DNA for gene conversion with class I molecules.

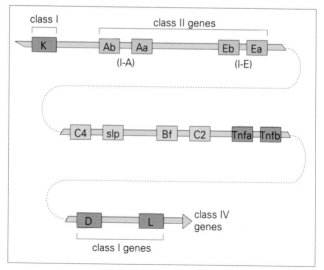

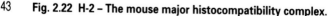

Fig. 2.22 H-2 – The mouse major histocompatibility complex.

HLA (Human Leucocyte Antigen) locus is the human major histo-compatibility complex, and is divided into 7 main regions, DP, DQ, DR, class III, B, C and A. It is thought that a number of class IV genes lie downstream of HLA-A. The overall layout is very similar to that of the mouse H-2 region.

HLA-A, -B and -C loci encode class I MHC molecules defined sero-logically, i.e. using monoclonal antibodies. The A and B loci show greatest polymorphism with 25 and 33 haplotypes respectively, whereas 11 have been defined at the -C locus.

HLA-DP, -DQ and -DR loci encode class II MHC molecules. Originally these were described as HLA-D specificities detected by their ability to stimulate allogeneic cells in a mixed lymphocyte cul-ture (MLC). Now the different molecules are defined serologically, although this can only be partly related to their HLA-D designation. DP and DQ each encode one pair of class II α and β chains, plus pseudogenes. The DR locus encodes one non-polymorphic α chain and 1 – 4 β chains depending on the individual haplotype.

HLA class III molecules are encoded between the class II loci and the class I loci. They include the C2 and factor B genes and the pseudoalleles for C4, C4F and C4S which determine the Rogers and Chido blood groups respectively. Genes for TNF-α, TNF-β and some heat shock proteins lie here.

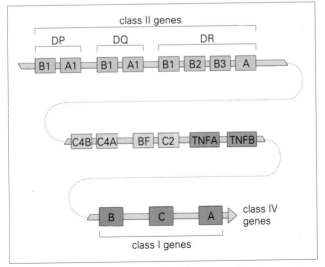

Fig. 2.23 HLA – The human major histocompatibility complex.   44

IMMUNE RECOGNITION BY T CELLS

MHC Restriction. T cells recognize antigen associated with particular MHC molecules. For example a T cell which recognizes an antigen associated with H-2K^b will not recognize it associated with H-2D^b or H-2K^k. Such interactions are MHC restricted. The basis of the observation is that T cells that interact with self MHC molecules are selectively expanded in the thymus, and are then primed to respond to antigen on APCs expressing these MHC molecules. Subsequently they will respond only to that antigen/MHC combination. Experimentally, it is possible to determine whether an immune interaction involves MHC molecules by seeing whether it is MHC restricted.

Class I/class II restriction refers to whether a particular group of T cells recognize antigen associated with MHC class I or class II molecules. In practice, CD8$^+$ cells are class I restricted, whereas CD4$^+$ cells are class II restricted.

CD4 and CD8 are functionally analagous molecules expressed on mature T cells. The cells have either CD4 or CD8 but not both. CD8 consists of two disulphide-linked transmembrane polyeptides, which can interact with the TCR on the T cells and which bind to a site in the α_3 domain of class I MHC molecules on the target cell (see below). This interaction contributes to the stabilization of the immune recognition complex. CD4 has a single transmembrane polypeptide chain and performs a similar function in interactions with MHC class II bearing

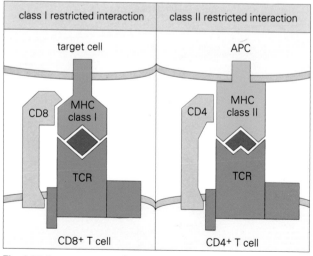

Fig. 2.24 Immune recognition by T cells.

APCs. These molecules also appear to become phosphorylated during T cell activation.

CD2 (Sheep erythrocyte receptor) is expressed on all T cells, and is involved in T cell activation. It has a single transmembrane polypeptide chain, which acts as a receptor for LFA-3. Interaction of CD2 with LFA-3 enhances the binding of the T cell to its target. T cells can be activated by crosslinking their CD2 molecules, but it is thought that the normal function is to amplify an activation signal initiated by the TCR/CD3 complex. Cell activation via CD2 causes phosphorylation of CD33 and CD37.

Lymphocyte functional antigens (LFA-1 – LFA-3) were originally identified as surface molecules involved in enhancing lymphocyte binding to other cells. LFA-1 is a member of the β_2 integrin family present on most leucocytes. It consists of two polypeptide chains (CD11a, CD18) which interact with the adhesion molecules ICAM-1 and ICAM-2. Lymphocyte activation enhances the affinity of LFA-1 thereby increasing the strength of lymphocyte binding. LFA-2 is CD2. LFA-3, the receptor for CD2, is widely distributed on many cell types, and contributes to lymphocyte activation by crosslinking CD2.

CD45 (Leucocyte common antigen) is present on all leucocytes and is produced in 6 different forms, using different combinations of exons. B cells express the highest molecular weight form. It is thought to be involved in the early stages of cell activation, by controlling phosphorylation of molecules such as CD4 and CD3.

adhesion molecule	structure	present on	ligands
LFA-1 (CD11a/CD18)	integrin	leucocytes	ICAM-1 ICAM-2
ICAM-1 (CD54)	5 domain Ig supergene family	activated T cells, vascular endothelium	LFA-1
CD2 (LFA-2)	2 domain Ig supergene family	T cells	LFA-3
LFA-3 (CD58)	2 domain Ig supergene family (2 forms differing in membrane anchorage)	wide distribution including thymic epithelium, endothelium, lymphocytes	CD2

Fig. 2.25 Auxillary molecules in immune recognition.

Immune Responses | 3

ADAPTIVE AND INNATE IMMUNITY

The immune response is mediated by a variety of cells and soluble factors, broadly divided according to whether they mediate adaptive (acquired) or innate (natural) immunity.

Adaptive (Acquired) immunity is specific for the inducing agent, and is marked by an enhanced response on repeated encounters with that agent. Thus the key features of the adaptive immune response are *memory* and *specificity*.

Innate (Natural) immunity depends on a variety of immunological effector mechanisms, which are neither specific for particular infectious agents nor improved by repeated encounters with the same agent. In practice, there is considerable overlap between these two types of immunity, since the adaptive immune system can direct elements of the innate system, such as phagocytes or complement. The principle elements of the innate immune system are outlined below and on the following pages.

Complement system is a group of serum molecules involved in the control of inflammation, removal of immune complexes and lysis of pathogens or cells sensitized with antibody.

Acute phase proteins describes those serum molecules which increase rapidly at the onset of infection. The most notable is C-reactive protein (CRP) which binds the C-protein of *Pneumococci* and facilitates their uptake by phagocytes.

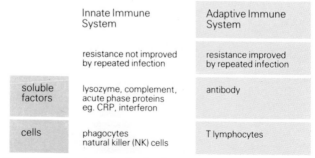

	Innate Immune System	Adaptive Immune System
	resistance not improved by repeated infection	resistance improved by repeated infection
soluble factors	lysozyme, complement, acute phase proteins eg. CRP, interferon	antibody
cells	phagocytes natural killer (NK) cells	T lymphocytes

Fig. 3.1 The innate and adaptive immune systems.

Interferons (IFNs) are a group of molecules which limit the spread of viral infections. There are three types, IFN-α and IFN-β produced by leucocytes and fibroblasts and IFN-γ produced by activated T cells. Interferons from activated or virally infected cells bind to receptors on nearby cells inducing them to make anti-viral proteins. IFN-α and IFN-β bind to one type of receptor, while IFN-γ binds to another. IFN-γ also has many other immunomodulatory functions.

Anti-viral proteins are molecules that are induced by IFNs, which limit viral replication. Many of them are produced in an inactive form, and are only activated by contact with virus or its products, such as double stranded RNA. Some, activated by an incoming virus, block the initiation of protein synthesis, whereas others lead to mRNA degradation.

Cell-mediated immunity and Humoral immunity are traditional ways of describing the different arms of the immune system. Antibody, complement and other soluble molecules constitute the humoral effector systems, whereas T cells, NK cells and phagocytes constitute the cellular effectors. With advances in our understanding of immune recognition, it is more useful to think in terms of the systems that recognize free antigens, and those that recognize cell-associated antigens. For example cytotoxic T cells can recognize antigens presented on cell membranes which have originated from within that cell, whereas antibody is particularly important in the recognition of free, extracellular antigens.

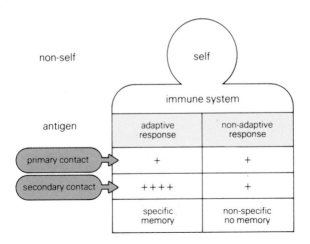

Fig. 3.2 Primary and secondary immune responses.

PHAGOCYTOSIS

Phagocytosis is the process by which cells engulf particles and microorganisms. The particles first attach to the cell membrane of the phagocytic cell, either by non-specific receptors such as the lectin-like receptors which bind bacterial carbohydrates, or by receptors for opsonins such as IgG and C3b. Then the cell extends pseudopodia around the particle and internalizes it. Anti-bacterial oxygen-dependent killing mechanisms are activated, and lysosomes fuse with the phagosome. The lysosomal enzymes damage and digest the phagocytosed material and digestion products are finally released.

Pinocytosis is phagocytosis on a small scale, in which cells take up small volumes of extracellular fluid.

Endocytosis is the term now commonly used for internalization of material by phagocytosis or pinocytosis.

Opsonization occurs when particles, microorganisms or immune complexes become coated with molecules which allow them to bind to receptors on phagocytes, thereby enhancing their uptake.

Opsonins are molecules which bind to particles to be phagocytosed and to receptors on phagocytes, so acting as a bridge

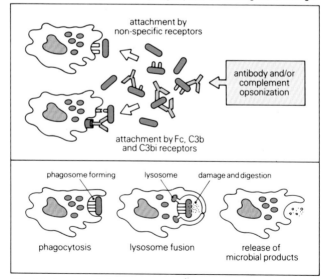

Fig. 3.3 Stages of phagocytosis.

between the two, e.g. IgG, C3b and C-reactive protein.

Immune adherence refers to the attachment of opsonized particles to phagocytes, effected by IgG and C3 products, binding to Fc and complement receptors (see pages 53 & 54).

Frustrated phagocytosis occurs when phagocytes attach to material which cannot be phagocytosed (e.g. basement membrane). The cells may release their lysosomal enzymes to the exterior (exocytosis). This process is thought to cause some of the damage in immune complex diseases.

Phagosomes are the membrane bound intracellular vesicles which contain phagocytosed materials.

Oxygen-dependent killing occurs within phagosomes and is activated via crosslinking of the phagocytes C3 and Fc receptors. Initially an enzyme in the phagosome membrane, reduces oxygen to superoxide (O_2^-), which can then give rise to hydroxyl radicals (OH^-), singlet oxygen ($O\cdot$) and hydrogen peroxide (H_2O_2).

Reactive oxygen intermediates (ROIs) refer to the labile products of the oxygen-dependent killing pathway (above) and which can damage endocytosed bacteria. Cells prevent damage to them-

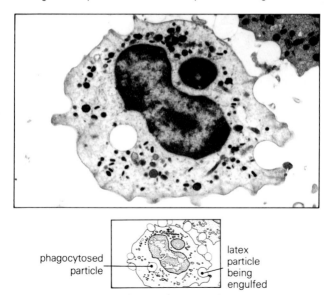

phagocytosed particle — latex particle being engulfed

Fig. 3.4 Phagocytosis of latex by a macrophage.

selves by redox pathways involving glutathione, but some bacteria deploy similar defences against ROIs.

Peroxidase present in lysosomes can enter the phagosome where, in the presence of H_2O_2, it converts halide ions into toxic halogen compounds (e.g. hypohalite). Endocytosed peroxidase or catalase can also perform this reaction.

Respiratory burst. Shortly after phagocytosing material, neutrophils and macrophages undergo a burst of activity, during which they increase their oxygen consumption. This is associated with increased activity of the hexose monophosphate shunt and production of H_2O_2 and $O_2 \cdot$.

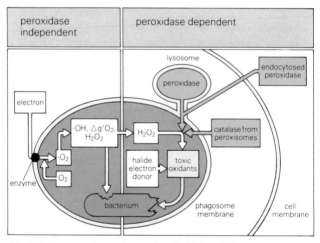

Fig. 3.5 Oxygen-dependent microbicidal activity.

Chemiluminescence is the production of light by chemical reactions. It occurs during the respiratory burst.

Lysosomes are organelles present in all cells. They contain enzymes, which in macrophages, damage and digest the phagocytosed material. Newly forming lysosomes are called 'primary' and mature lysosomes are 'secondary'.

Phagolysosomes are formed by the fusion of phagosomes and lysosome. Immediately after phagosome/lysosome fusion there is a brief rise in the pH of the phagolysosome and neutral proteases and cationic proteins are active. Subsequently the pH falls and acid proteases become active.

Granules are specialized lysosomes of granulocytes which contain various bactericidal proteins. Each type of granule has a particular set of proteins. For example, neutrophil myeloperoxidase is in the primary (azurophilic) granules whereas lactoferrin is in the secondary (neutrophil specific) granules.

Granule and lysosome contents include:

Lysozyme (muramidase), an enzyme which digests a bond in the cell wall proteoglycan of some Gram-positive bacteria. It is secreted constitutively by neutrophils and some macrophages and is present in many of the body's secretions.

Cationic proteins, found in neutrophil granules and in some macrophages, damage the outer lipid bilayer of some Gram-negative bacteria under alkaline conditions. This activity is produced by a number of molecules some of which (e.g. cathepsin G) are enzymically active.

Acid proteases, active at acid pH, include enzymes such as glycosidase, nuclease, lipase and acid phosphatase.

Neutral proteases, active near pH 7, include enzymes such as collagenase, elastase and some cathepsins.

Lactoferrin, found in neutrophil granules, binds tightly to iron, thus depriving bacteria of this essential element. Neutrophils loaded with iron are inefficient at destroying bacteria.

Macrophage activation refers to the enhanced anti-microbial (or anti-tumour) activity seen in response to stimulation by lymphokines, complement fragments etc. Activated cells secrete more enzymes, produce more superoxide and express more Fc and C3b receptors.

Chediak-Higashi syndrome is a condition with impaired phagocyte responses to chemoattractants and reduced killing of phagocytosed bacteria. The disorder appears to lie in the cytoskeleton.

Chronic Granulomatous Disease (CGD) is a genetic defect where oxygen-dependent bacterial killing is impaired and mononuclear cells accumulate at sites of chronic inflammation, forming granulomas.

Leucocyte adhesion deficiency (Lad) syndrome is characterized by poor neutrophil localization into tissues and impaired phagocytosis. It is due to a failure to produce CD18, the common β chain of LFA-1 and complement receptors CR3 and CR4.

COMPLEMENT RECEPTORS

There are four different kinds of receptor for activated C3 (CR1 - CR4) and three of these act as receptors for immune complexes on cells of the mononuclear phagocyte lineage.

CR1 (CD35) is a transmembrane protein consisting of a single polypeptide which occurs on phagocytic cells where it acts as a receptor for immune complexes. It can also facilitate breakdown of the bound C3b. It is present on erythrocytes in man, where it facilitates transport of complexes to phagocytic cells in spleen and liver. It is also present on some lymphocytes, although its function on these cells is less certain.

CR2 (CD21) is structurally similar to CR1, but occurs only on B cells and follicular dendritic cells. It is thought be involved in the uptake of complexes to germinal centres and in the development of B cell memory.

CR3 (CD11b/CD18) is a member of the integrin family of molecules, consisting of an α and β chain. It is expressed on mononuclear phagocytes, neutrophils and NK cells, where it facilitates the uptake of immune complexes with bound C3d. It may also be involved in leucocyte migration into tissues.

CR4 (CD11c/CD18), also called p150,95, is an integrin which has a common β chain with CR3, and similar functions, although it is particularly highly expressed on tissue macrophages.

C1q receptor (C1qR) is only partially characterized, but appears to be involved in the uptake of complexes carrying C1q.

receptor	specificity	present on:	function in:
CR1	C3b, C4b	erythrocytes lymphocytes phagocytes	transport of complexes ? complex uptake
CR2	iC3b, C3d	B cells follicular dendritic cells	development of B cell memory
CR3	iC3b	phagocytes LGLs	uptake of complexes cytotoxicity
CR4	iC3b	phagocytes LGL's	uptake of complexes cytotoxicity

53   **Fig. 3.6 Receptors for activated C3.**

Fc RECEPTORS

There are three well defined receptors for IgG on phagocytic cells which facilitate the uptake of immune complexes, and allow cytotoxic cells to interact with targets sensitized with antibody. These are designated FcγRI - FcγRIII. Less well defined receptors for different antibody classes are found on subpopulations of lymphocytes, and are thought to be involved in controlling production of different antibody isotypes. In addition two receptors for IgE have been described, FcεRI and FcεRII, the first having a role in the control of inflammatory mediator release, the second having an immunoregulatory role.

FcγRI (CD64) is a high affinity IgG receptor capable of binding monomeric antibody. It is a characteristic marker of mononuclear phagocytes but may also be expressed on activated neutrophils. It is thought to be involved in the uptake of immune complexes.

FcγRII (CD32) is a low affinity receptor present on mononuclear phagocytes, neutrophils, eosinophils, platelets and B cells. On phagocytic cells it appears to facilitate phagocytosis of large complexes, but on B cells it is thought to be involved in control of antibody production. Crosslinking of the surface antibody and Fc receptors on B cells leads to downregulation of the B cell. Activation of platelets by immune complexes bound to their Fc receptors can lead to degranulation with release of inflammatory mediators.

FcγRIII (CD16) is a low affinity IgG receptor which occurs in two forms. On LGLs it is a transmembrane glycoprotein (CD16-2) which can crosslink the cells to target cells sensitized with antibody. Engagement of this receptor on LGLs leads to cell activation. On macrophages and neutrophils it is a phosphotidyl inositol-linked receptor, attached to the membrane where it can bind immune complexes, but cannot signal cell activation.

FcεRI is a high affinity IgE receptor found on mast cells and basophils. These cells can take up monomeric IgE, which sensitizes them. When the particular IgE-binding antigen crosslinks these receptors, it leads to degranulation, with release of histamine and other inflammatory mediators.

FcεRII (CD23) is a low affinity IgE receptor present on some B cells, thought to have an immunoregulatory function. A soluble form of the receptor acts as a signalling molecule between lymphocytes. It is also present on eosinophils where it may allow them to engage parasites (e.g. schistosomes) coated with IgE.

CYTOTOXICITY

Cytotoxicity is general term for the ways in which lymphocytes, mononuclear phagocytes and granulocytes can kill target cells. This kind of interaction is important in the destruction of cells which have become infected with viruses, or intracellular microorganisms, which they are unable to eliminate.

T cell mediated cytotoxicity involves recognition of antigen fragments associated with MHC class I molecules (usually) on the surface of the target cell, and is effected by $CD8^+$ Tc cells. The attacking cell orientates its granules towards the target and releases the contents, including perforin and granzymes, at the junction between the cells. target cell death occurs by apoptosis.

Perforin is a pore-forming molecule related to complement C9, which polymerizes on the target cell membrane to form channels.

Granzymes are serine proteases found in the granules of cytotoxic T cells, which could damage target cells.

Apoptosis is a form of programmed cell death, in which the cell and its DNA both fragment.

Antibody-Dependent Cell-Mediated Cytotoxicity (ADCC) involves recognition of target cells coated with antibody. This may be effected by LGLs, macrophages or granulocytes, using their Fcγ receptors. The mechanism of cytotoxic damage depends on the

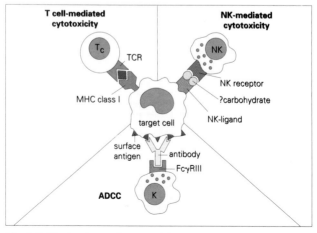

Fig. 3.7 Mechanisms of cytotoxicity.

effector cell - macrophages can release enzymes and reactive oxygen intermediates, whereas LGLs use perforins and cytokines.

NK cell-mediated cytotoxicity is mediated by large granular lymphocytes, which engage their targets via a partly defined receptor, unrelated to the TCR. There is some evidence that the ligand on the target cell is carbohydrate, and the mechanism of cytotoxic damage is thought to be similar to those used by cytotoxic T cells.

Eosinophil-mediated cytotoxicity Eosinophils are only weakly phagocytic, and are less efficient than neutrophils and macrophages at destroying endocytosed pathogens. However, they can exocytose their granule contents releasing those factors which are most effective at damaging certain large parasites. The granule contents include phosphatases, aryl-sulphatase and histaminase, in addition to those listed below.

Major Basic Protein (MBP) is a highly cationic protein forming a major component of the crystalloid core of eosinophil granules. It is solubilized before secretion and can damage parasites.

Eosinophil Cationic Protein (ECP) is highly basic, zinc containing ribonuclease which binds avidly to negatively charges surfaces and is particularly effective at damaging the tegument of schistosomes.

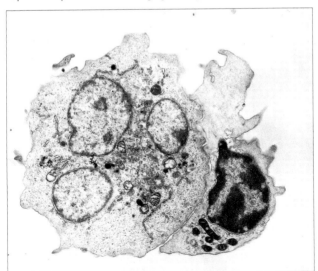

Fig. 3.8 Electronmicrograph of a K cell (right) engaging a target cell (left). x2500. Courtesy of Mr P. Penfold.

ANTIBODY RESPONSE

Following injection of an antigen, an antibody response develops which may be divided into four phases: a lag phase in which no antibody is detected, followed by a phase in which the antibody titres rise logarithmically, then plateau and decline, as the antibodies are catabolized or cleared as complexes.

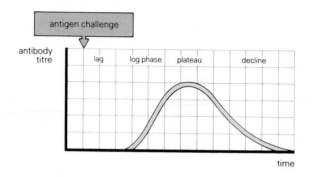

Fig. 3.9 Graph showing the four phases of a primary antibody response.

Primary and Secondary antibody responses. The quality of the antibody response following the second (secondary) encounter with antigen varies from that following the first (primary) contact. The primary response has a longer lag phase, reaches a lower plateau and declines more quickly than the secondary response. IgM is a major component of the primary response and is produced before IgG, whereas IgG is the main class represented in the secondary response. During their development some B cells switch from IgM production to other classes and this is the basis of the change in antibody isotype seen in the secondary response. Differences between the primary and secondary response are most noticeable when T dependent antigens are used, but the route of antigen entry and the way it is presented to T and B cells also affect the development of the response and the classes of antibody produced.

Prime and Challenge are terms used to describe the administration of antigen either *in vivo* or to cells *in vitro*. The first administration is priming; it may be insufficient to engender a measurable response, but can still produce memory or an enhanced secondary response. The term challenge is used loosely for any procedure which induces and immune response.

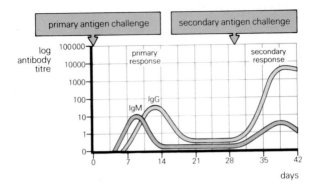

Fig. 3.10 Primary and secondary antibody responses.

Affinity maturation describes the finding that the average affinity of the induced antibodies increases in the secondary response. The effect is largely confined to IgG and is most marked when a low antigen dose is given in the secondary injection. Low levels of antigen bind preferentially to high affinity B cell clones and activate them - there is insufficient antigen to activate low affinity clones. The underlying cellular basis, is the change in the affinity of B cell clones caused by somatic hypermutation of the antibody genes. This accompanies, but is not dependent on, class switching. It does not occur in the response to T-independent antigens, which are predominantly IgM antibodies. Therefore the process is thought to be mediated by T cells.

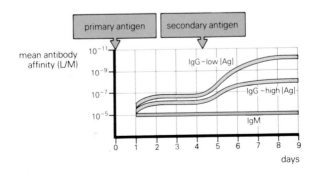

Fig. 3.11 Affinity maturation.

CELL COOPERATION IN THE IMMUNE RESPONSE

Cooperation between cells involved in immune responses occurs at many levels. Phagocytes and APCs can take up antigen in the periphery and transport it to secondary lymphoid tissues (spleen, lymph nodes etc). Antigen presenting cells and B cells can internalize antigen, process it and present it in association with MHC class II molecules to $CD4^+$ T_H cells. Cytokines produced by activated T cells can stimulate B cell growth and differentiation into plasma cells. Other cytokines can also activate T_C cells APCs and mononuclear phagocytes. Antibodies released by the B cells, can bind to receptors on phagocytes, thereby facilitating uptake of antigen. IgG antibodies allow LGLs (K cells) to recognize target cells coated with antibody, and IgE antibodies can sensitize mast cells and basophils to release their inflammatory mediators when they bind specific antigen. Cytokines and antibodies are soluble mediators of cell cooperation, but leucocytes also interact directly with each other. The most important direct interaction is that involving MHC molecules/antigenic peptides contacting the T cell receptor. But other interactions, for example CD2/LFA-3 or ICAM-1/LFA-1 are essential for cellular cooperation.

Antigen processing Antigens encountering the immune system often require processing before they can be recognized by lymphocytes (particularly so for T cells). The process involves partial degradation of the antigen. This may occur in phagolysosomes of mononuclear phagocytes, or at the surface of specialized APCs such as dendritic cells.

Antigen presentation is the process by which antigen is presented to lymphocytes in a form they can recognize. Most $CD4^+$ T_H cells must be presented with antigen on MHC class II molecules, while $CD8^+$ T_C cells only recognize antigen on class I MHC molecules. The way in which an antigen is processed and the type of MHC molecule it associates with, determines which T cells will recognize it, whether the antigen is immunogenic or tolerogenic and affects the type of immune response generated.

Costimulation. Most immune responses are initiated by antigen triggering B cells or T cells. However, cellular activation also requires other signals. These may be delivered via other surface molecules (e.g. intercellular adhesion molecules) or by cytokines. This is sometimes called the two-signal hypothesis, in which antigen provides the first signal and the other costimulatory interactions provide the second signal. Cells which only receive a first signal may become anergic (tolerant) to their particular antigen.

Cytokines (lymphokines) are a group of molecules, other than antibodies, produced by leucocytes which are involved in signalling between cells of the immune system. The group includes the interleukins, the interferons, the tumour necrosis factors (TNF) and the colony stimulating factors (CSF). The term lymphokines was originally used for those cytokines produced by lymphocytes.

T cell help describes the cooperative interactions involving TH cells, particularly in the production of the antibody response. To generate an antibody response to Tdep antigens requires cooperation between B cells and T cells. B cells bind to their specific antigen via their surface Ig and internalize it. They can process and present the antigen in association with MHC class II molecules for recognition by TH cells. The T cells in turn deliver costimulatory signals to the B cells and release cytokines, including IL-4, IL-5 and IL-6, which promote B cell division and differentiation.

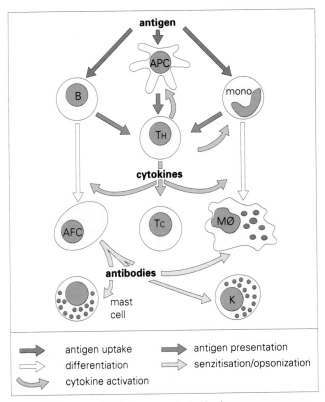

Fig. 3.12 Cooperation between cells in the immune response.

ANTIGEN PRESENTATION

Antigens are taken up by antigen-presenting cells in a variety of ways. B cells use surface antibody to bind and internalize their specific antigen. This is partly degraded (processed) and returned to the cell surface, associated with MHC class II molecules for recognition by T cells. Theoretically B cells can endocytose and present any antigen, but in practice they selectively concentrate only their own specific antigen, in sufficient quantities. Mononuclear phagocytes endocytose opsonized particles via their Fc and C3 receptors, which are broken down in phagolysosomes. However, this pathway for antigen-breakdown intersects the intracellular pathway for production of MHC class II molecules, and antigen fragments are transferred to the MHC molecules. The way in which dendritic cells handle antigen is less well understood: they may endocytose and degrade sufficient material themselves, or be capable of taking up antigens that have been degraded by other cells, or may partially proteolyse antigens at the cell surface.

Intermolecular help refers to the way in which B cells can take up antigenic particles carrying several different antigens (e.g. a virus). They can then process and present the entire set of antigens and present them to T cells. They receive T cell help from T cells specific for antigens they themselves do not recognize. For example, a B cell specific for flu virus haemagglutinin can internalize the virus and present it to neuraminidase specific T cells.

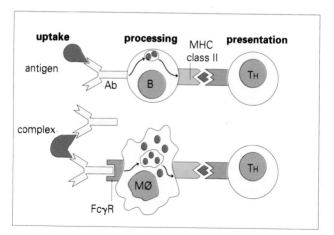

Fig. 3.13 Mechanisms of antigen uptake, processing and presentation by APCs.

Antigen processing is the cellular action involved in the degradation of antigen and association with MHC molecules. Blocking the degradative pathways renders cells unable to process and present most antigens. Different cell types have different capacities to degrade antigens and hence in their ability to stimulate T cells. There appear to be two distinct pathways for processing, used by MHC class I and class II molecules.

Class I and Class II pathways. Antigens synthesized within a cell, such as viral polypeptides, associate preferentially with MHC class I molecules. This occurs as the class I molecules are synthesized, and the association with antigen peptides helps to stabilize the class I α chain and its association with β_2-microglobulin. After synthesis these class I molecules are moved from the Golgi apparatus to the cell surface, where they may present any bound antigen to CD8$^+$ T cells. By contrast, antigens that have been endocytosed by a cell, such as immune complexes associate preferentially with MHC class II molecules. It is thought that the invariant chain Ii which is present on newly synthesized class II molecules is exchanged for antigen, in an endosomal compartment, before the class II molecule is transported to the cell surface.

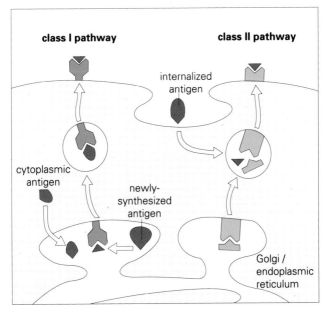

Fig. 3.14 Class I and Class II pathways of antigen presentation.

CYTOKINES

Cytokines, released by leucocytes and sometimes other cells, are very important in controlling the development of the immune response. They modulate the differentiation and division of haemopoietic stem cells and the activation of lymphocytes and phagocytes. Others can act as cytotoxins and it is now thought that the balances between help and suppression, tolerance and reaction, and antibody and cell-mediated immunity are all affected by cytokines. Many cytokines have more than one action (pleiotropy) and different cells produce different blends of cytokines. TH cells are particularly important sources of these mediators.

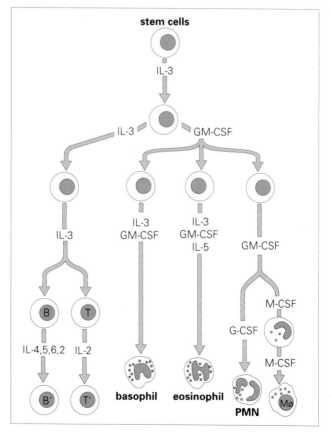

Fig. 3.15 Control of differentiation by CSFs.

Autocrine and Paracrine actions. Most cytokines act on cells other than those that produce them (paracrine action), but some can also stimulate the cell that produced them (autocrine action).

Synergy refers to the observation that combinations of cytokines can often produce effects which are more than additive, or generate responses which neither one alone can do. Sometimes one cytokine induces the receptors for another on a cell, in other cases a cell requires independent triggering by two mediators.

Colony Stimulating Factors (CSFs) control the differentiation of haemopoietic stem cells, both in the bone marrow and in the periphery (see opposite). This group consists of granulocyte, macrophage and granulocyte/macrophage colony stimulating factors (G-CSF, M-CSF and GM-CSF respectively). These promote the development of their specific subsets of leucocytes. In addition IL-3, IL-5 and erythropoietin are functionally members of this group. IL-3 promotes the differentiation of all the leucocyte lineages, whereas IL-5 is necessary for eosinophil development. Erythropoietin promotes the expansion of erythroid colony forming units.

Interferon-γ (IFN-γ) is released by antigen-activated T cells. In addition to its anti-viral effects, IFN-γ can enhance MHC class I and II expression on B cells and macrophages, and at higher levels induces class II on many tissue cells to enhance antigen presentation. It increases IL-2 receptors on Tc cells, enhances cytotoxic activity of LGLs and promotes B cell differentiation. IFN-γ is the principle cytokine responsible for 'Macrophage Arming Factor' (MAF) activity which increases FcγR expression and induces the respiratory burst, thereby enhancing their ability to destroy pathogens.

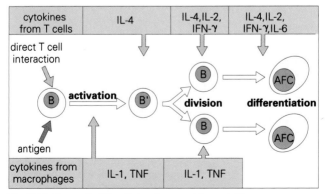

Fig. 3.16 Control of B cell development by cytokines. 64

Migration Inhibition Factor (MIF) is a partly characterized cytokine released by activated T cells which inhibits macrophage migration and is important in causing the accumulation of these cells at site of inflammation.

Tumour Necrosis Factor (TNF) and Lymphotoxin (LT) are structurally related cytokines encoded within the MHC. Lymphotoxin, released by Tc cells, is now called TNF-β, whereas the original TNF, released by activated macrophages and several other cell types, is TNF-α. In addition to its cytotoxic activity TNF-α enhances the adhesiveness of vascular endothelium for lymphocytes,

cytokine	source	target	principle effects
IL-1α	macrophage fibroblast lymphocytes	lymphocytes macrophages other	lymphocyte costimulation activation of phagocytes prostaglandin production numerous effects
IL-1β	epithelial cells astrocytes		
IL-2	T cells	T cells LGLs (B cells)	T cell growth & activation
IL-3	T cells mast cells	stem cells	promotes haemopoietic cell production
IL-4	T cells bone marrow stroma	B cells	early activation
IL-5	T cells macrophages	T cells B cells(mouse)	division & differentiation
IL-6	macrophages fibroblasts T cells	B cells T cells hepatocytes	B cell differentiation acute phase protein induction
IL-7	bone marrow stroma	lymphocytes	division
IL-8	fiboblasts monocytes endothelium	monocytes T cells neutrophils	chemotaxis
IL-9	T cells	T cells	division
IL-10	T cells	lymphocytes	?

Fig. 3.17 The interleukins.

thereby promoting transendothelial migration. The induction of acute phase protein synthesis by liver in response to TNF is probably mediated via IL-6. TNF also causes the mobilization of fat which is partly responsible for the wasting (cachexia) seen in some chronic diseases. It also synergizes with IFN-γ in many of its actions, such as MHC induction, and the promotion LGL and macrophage activation.

Interleukins (IL-1 – IL-10) are a series of diverse cytokines; most newly discovered cytokines are placed in this series. Their principle properties are indicated opposite. IL-1 has many similar effects to TNF, including enhancing leucocyte/endothelial cell adhesion and inducing acute phase proteins. It can also act on hypothalamic centres to induce fever and sleep. It acts on fibroblasts, osteoclasts and chondrocytes to produce prostaglandins and promote tissue remodelling. IL-1 induces IL-2 receptors on T cells and therefore acts as a costimulator in T cell activation. IL-2 is an essential T cell growth factor (TCGF) required for division of antigen-activated T cells. Activated B cells also express IL-2 receptors. IL-3 is a pan-specific haemopoietin (see above). IL-4 – IL-7 are B cell growth and differentiation factors released by TH cells. IL-4 is essential for early B cell activation and clonal expansion, whereas IL-5 and IL-6 promote their subsequent differentiation into antibody secreting cells. IL-4 tends to promote class-switching to IgG2a (in mouse) whereas IFN-γ promotes IgG1 production. IL-8 is a chemotactic factor released by activated monocytes which is chemotactic for neutrophils and basophils and causes monocytes to adhere to endothelium. IL-9 and IL-10 are growth factors.

B Cell Stimulating Factors (BSFs) is an older nomenclature used for IL-4 to IL-6. IL-4 is B cell growth factor type I (BCGF-I), IL-5 is BCGF-II and IL-6, originally identified as IFN-β$_2$ is a B cell differentiation factor (BCDF).

Cytokine receptors determine the responsiveness of a cell to particular cytokines. Receptors for IL-1, TNF and the interferons are widely distributed. The high affinity IL-2 receptor, consists of two polypeptide chains and is recognizable by the TAC monoclonal antibody (CD25). It appears on antigen-activated T cells, for a limited period, thereby controlling T cell division, but expression wanes if the T cell is not restimulated with antigen. Expression of receptors for IL-4 - IL-6 occurs on activated B cells in an analagous fashion. Receptors for the colony-stimulating factors appear during haemopoietic cell differentiation on the appropriate developing cells.

IMMUNE RESPONSE GENES

Responder and non-responder. Inbred strains of animals produce a characteristic level of immune response to injected antigens. Strains which produce high levels are responders, others are low responders. The status depends mostly on the immune response genes of the MHC and varies with different antigens.

Immune response (Ir) genes. A large number of genes determine the level of an immune response to an antigen. Ir genes control antigen processing and presentation, cell cooperation, the repertoire of antigen receptors, production of cytokines and their receptors and the processes of cellular activation. The most important Ir genes encode class II MHC molecules, which control the way in which each antigen is presented.

Repertoire is the sum total of antigen receptors produced by the immune system. The initial repertoire is partly determined by the genes of the TCR and antibody H and L chains.

Clonal restriction. This refers to an immune response produced by a limited number of clones. For example, the primary immune response to phosphoryl choline in Ig^a haplotype mice is predominantly generated by B cells expressing the T15 idiotype. T cell responses can also be clonally restricted with selective use of particular T cell receptor V genes. This is related to selective antigen presentation by particular MHC molecules.

Holes (in the repertoire) are a way of explaining the non-responder status of an animal because it lacks some particular antigen receptor. In practice this effect is more often due to lack of an appropriate MHC molecule.

macrophage function	low responder	high responder
1. antigen uptake	+++	+
2. lysosomal enzyme activity	+++	+
3. intracellular degradation of antigen	+++	+
4. surface persistence of antigen	+	+++

Fig. 3.18 Macrophage functions in high and low responder mice.

Biozzi mice are strains genetically inbred to give high or low antibody responses to an antigen (originally sheep erythrocytes). At least ten separate non-MHC gene loci control responsiveness in these animals. The high and low responder strains differ in the way their macrophages handle antigens - low responders degrade antigen quickly and do not present it.

Genetic restriction describes the finding that cells cooperate most effectively when they share an MHC haplotype. The effect is seen in macrophage/T cell interactions, in T cell/B cell cooperation and in Tc mediated destruction of infected target cells - all situations where antigen presentation to T cells is occurring. The basis of the observation is that a population of T cells educated in the thymus to interact with their own MHC molecules and primed by APCs expressing those molecules, will subsequently only interact with cells expressing that particular set (haplotypes) of molecules. This effect is illustrated below. Irradiated (X) animals of MHC haplotype CxD were reconstituted with T cells primed to carrier (BGG') and B cells primed to hapten (DNP'). After challenge with BGG-DNP the response to DNP was measured. A response is obtained where T and B cells share at least one haplotype (C or D).

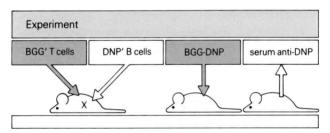

experiment	T cells	B cells	recipient	response
1	C	C	CxD	+
2	D	D	CxD	+
3	C	D	CxD	−
4	D	C	CxD	−
5	CxD	D	CxD	+

Fig. 3.19 Genetic restriction in T/B cooperation.

IMMUNOREGULATION

The immune response is regulated primarily by antigen, and secondarily by interactions between lymphocytes, APCs and their products, including antibody and cytokines. Antigen is the primary initiator of immune responses, since the first signal required to trigger lymphocytes is antigen or antigen/MHC. Indeed the immune system may be viewed as a single homeostatic unit for the elimination of antigen. In this view antigen initiates an immune response, which eliminates that antigen, and the immune system then returns to the resting state. The essential role of antigen is seen at the cellular level. In the example below antigen/MHC triggers T cell activation, and expression of receptors for cytokines (e.g. IL-2) required for T cell division. T cell help causes B cells to produce specific antibody, leading to elimination of the antigen. With the disappearance of antigen, there is no longer any first activation signal for the B cells. Likewise the lack of an antigen/MHC activation signal for the T cells causes them to lose their cytokine receptors and stop cytokine production. The immune system then falls back to the resting state.

Antibody feedback. Antibody regulates its own production in several ways: 1) Binding to antigen and thus preventing the antigen from activating lymphocytes, as indicated above; 2) Binding to Fc receptors on B cells, which in the presence of antigen causes crosslinking of the Fc receptors and surface Ig. This delivers an inhibtory signal to the cells; 3) By promoting immune complex formation and localization of antigen to germinal centres, it induces B cell memory.

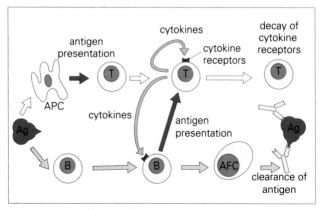

69   **Fig. 3.20 Immunoregulation.**

Immunoregulation falls into three classes:

Antigen specific interactions are confined to cells which bind a particular antigen, and must be mediated therefore by antigen receptors - see for example (2) above.

Idiotype specific interactions are confined to cells and antibodies expressing particular idiotypes on their antigen receptors. For example during a response to a particular antigen, one particular group of lymphocytes carrying a particular idiotype may be expanded or deleted.

Non-specific interactions affect lymphocytes regardless of their idiotype or antigen specificity. Cytokine-mediated and neuro-endocrine regulation is non-specific. However in practice the structural organization of the lymphoid system means that non-specific signals are localized in their effects.

Suppression. A regulatory group of T cells (T suppressors, Ts) are thought to modulate the activity of other lymphocytes. Early experiments indicated that Ts cells were CD8$^+$, but no specific marker for these cells has been identified and CD4$^+$ cells can also sometimes be suppressive. This is, therefore, a functional definition. Suppression is an active process and can be distinguished from tolerance by transferring the suppression with T cells. The cellular basis for this type of immunoregulation is obscure but may involve some or all of the following mechanisms: 1) A specific cytostatic action of CD8$^+$ Tc cells; 2) Passive blocking of lymphocyte activation by sequestering essential cytokines required for cell division; 3) Secretion of immunosuppressive molecules such as prostaglandins; 4) An immunoregulatory effect caused by the local production of specific sets of cytokines, causing cells to switch between different modes of immune response; 5) Induction of clonal anergy due to the Ts cells supplying an activation signal, but not the required costimulatory signals or cytokines.

Contrasuppression is the action of a group of T cells which render TH cells resistant to suppression. The nature of the cells and indeed this whole area is highly controversial.

Suppressor macrophages. This is a functional description of the action of macrophages in some experimental systems. The suppression is non-specific and is often mediated by cytokines or prostaglandins.

IDIOTYPE NETWORKS

Anti-idiotypes (anti-Id) are antibodies which react with epitopes on the V region of antibodies or the TCR.

Network hypothesis is a theory that lymphocytes may be regulated in their interactions by recognition of the idiotypes on the antigen receptors of other cells, or by idiotype-bearing antibodies. For example, an anti-idiotypic antibody could cause the down-regulation of the set of B cells expressing the idiotype. The theory does not make predictions as to whether the interactions will be enhancing or suppressive. An idiotype network is illustrated below where antigen (Ag) induces an idiotype (Ab1) which in turn induces anti-Ids (Ab2) and anti-anti-Ids (Ab3). The physiological relevance of such regulation is doubtful.

Internal image anti-idiotype is an anti-idiotype which recognizes an idiotype to an external antigen, and structurally resembles the external antigen, e.g. the upper Ab2, below.

Parallel sets are antibodies which share an idiotope but are directed towards different antigens. According to the network hypothesis they may be regulated concommitantly.

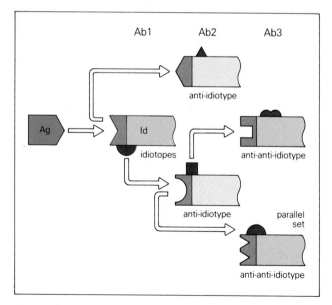

71   **Fig. 3.21 Jerne's Network hypothesis.**

NEUROENDOCRINE REGULATION OF IMMUNE RESPONSES

There is evidence that neurological events can affect immunological functions, either directly or via the endocrine system.

Innervation of lymphoid tissues. Thymus, spleen and lymph nodes all receive sympathetic noradrenergic innervation. These control blood flow through the lymphoid tissues, thus affecting lymphocyte traffic. However, fibres also run between the lymphocytes and appear to form junctions with individual cells. Denervation of lymphoid tissues can modulate immune responses.

Pituitary/adrenal axis. Stress can induce release of adrenocorticotrophic hormone from the pituitary. This induces release of glucocorticoids, which are immunosuppressive. Lymphocytes also produce ACTH in response to corticotrophin releasing factor (CRF). In addition the adrenal medulla releases catecholamines which can alter leucocyte migration patterns and lymphocyte responsiveness.

Endocrine and neuropeptide regulation. Lymphocytes carry receptors for many hormones, including insulin, thyroxine, growth hormone and somatostatin. These hormones, as well as enkephalins and endorphins released during stress, modulate T and B cell functions in complex ways, depending on the level of mediators.

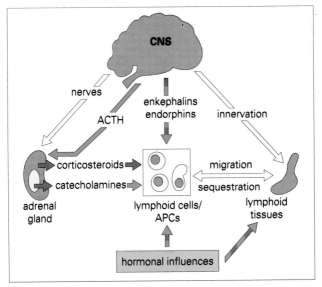

Fig. 3.22 Neuroendocrine regulation of immune responses.

IMMUNOSUPPRESSION

Immunosuppression describes measures used to reduce immune responses, particularly in transplantation surgery to prevent graft rejection and in the control of autoimmune diseases. Most measures are not antigen-specific although some drugs have greater effects on the immune system than other tissues.

Steroids, including glucocorticosteroids, corticosteroids and synthetic steroids such as dexamethasone have numerous immunosuppressive and anti-inflammatory effects, macrophages being particularly sensitive. They inhibit arachidonic acid release and hence reduce eicosanoid production They also reduce secretion of neutral proteases and IL-1. Steroids interfere with antigen presentation, inhibit the primary antibody response and reduce the numbers of circulating T cells.

Azathioprine and 6-mercaptopurine are purine analogues which act on small lymphocytes and dividing cells, thereby blocking development of effector cells. Monocytes are reduced, and K cell activity is also inhibited.

Cyclophosphamide and chlorambucil are alkylating agents which damage DNA and prevent its replication. They act primarily on lymphocytes and strongly inhibit antibody responses, but have little effect on phagocytes. Experimentally, cyclophosphamide prevents B cells from regenerating their receptors.

Cyclosporin-A is a fungal metabolite which interferes with early events in lymphocyte activation and transformation. It does not affect lymphoblasts, nor is it anti-mitotic or cytotoxic. It acts primarily on T cells and is the drug of first choice in transplantation surgery.

Fk506 is a bacterial compound which prevents T cell activation and mitogenesis, possibly by blocking IL-2 production. Its mode of action is thought to resemble that of cyclosporin-A.

Anti-lymphocyte globulin is an antibody raised to lymphocytes, which has been used in tissue grafting in man. It has been superceded by monoclonal antibodies.

Irradiation by x-rays given either locally or generally causes DNA damage and is immunosuppressive. Small resting lymphocytes and some APCs are highly radiosensitive, whereas suppressor cells are more resistant, although very high doses will eliminate all lymphocytes including stem cells.

IMMUNOPOTENTIATION

Biological Response Modifiers (BRM) are compounds which modify an immune response, usually enhancing it. This includes immunopotentiating bacterial products, chemicals such as polynucleotides, physiologically active molecules including cytokines, as well as the true adjuvants which are administered together with antigen. A number of these substances have been used in an attempt to potentiate immune reactions in cancer patients and immunodeficiency. Bacterial products include:

BCG (Bacillus Calmette Guerin) a live non-virulent strain of *Mycobacterium bovis* which is used in vaccines for immunization against tuberculosis.

Muramyl dipeptide (MDP) is the smallest adjuvant active part of BCG extractable from the cell wall.

Corynebacterium parvum induces lymphoid hyperplasia and activates macrophages.

Bordetella pertussis produces a lymphocytosis promoting factor (LPF) which is a T cell mitogen and an immunostimulant. *B. pertussis* causes whooping cough.

Adjuvants. These are compounds which enhance the immune response when administered with antigen, thereby producing higher antibody titres and prolonged production. The distinction between primary and secondary immune responses becomes blurred when adjuvants are used. Common adjuvants are:

Complete and Incomplete Freund's Adjuvant (CFA & IFA) is a stable water in oil emulsion which forms an antigen depot. The Complete adjuvant contains killed *M. tuberculosis*.

Alum where the antigen is coprecipitated with alum.

Thymic hormones are factors produced by the thymus which assist T cell development in the thymus and their maintenance in the periphery. They include thymosin, thymopoietin, thymostimulin and Facteur thymique serique (FTS).

Lymphokine Activated Killer (LAK) cells are syngeneic cytotoxic T cells generated *in vitro* by treating an individual's cells with cytokines, such as IL-2 and IFN-γ. They are sometimes reinfused into patients for cancer immunotherapy.

TOLERANCE

Tolerance is the acquisition of non-responsiveness to a molecule recognized by the immune system. Whether a molecule induces an immune response or tolerance is largely determined by the way in which it is first presented to the immune system.

Neonatal tolerance. Neonatal animals are very susceptible to the induction of tolerance due to the general immaturity of their immune systems. Consequently, tolerance induced at this stage of life is very persistent.

Self tolerance. It is observed that animals generally tolerate their own tissues – if they do not autoimmune disease may result. Self tolerance is thought to be due primarily to clonal abortion of cells in the neonatal period. As new mature lymphocytes develop they too are aborted just when they are most susceptible to tolerization (See education of T cells).

Superantigens are antigens which associate particularly effectively with MHC molecules, and which can induce clonal deletion of T cells which recognize them. Potentially they can modulate the repertoire of T cells generated.

Tolerization is the process by which tolerance can be induced in animals by administration of antigen in tolerizing regimes. Either B cells or T cells (or both) can become tolerant to a molecule, and since most antibody responses require T/B cooperation, tolerance in either cell population will produce overall tolerance.

B cell tolerance. In general, immature cells are more susceptible to tolerance induction than mature cells, and can be tolerized by smaller doses of tolerogens. The dose of antigen and the way it is presented are critical. Pathways to B cell tolerance are shown below.

Clonal deletion is tolerance induced by the specific elimination of clones of antigen-reactive cells. Where reactive B cells are present, but unable to respond due to lack of T cell help, this is a functional deletion. Since potentially reactive B cells are often found in tolerant animals, this idea has become modified to the concept of clonal abortion.

Clonal abortion/Clonal anergy is similar to clonal deletion, except that the antigen-reactive cells are not eliminated. They are still present but are rendered inactive.

Antibody forming cell blockade. Very large amounts of T-independent antigens may interfere with antibody secretion, although it is very difficult to tolerize AFCs.

T cell tolerance. T cells are more easily tolerized than B cells. Once established the duration of T cell tolerance in an animal is usually longer than that of the B cells. Immature T cells may be deleted during thymic development. Mature T cells can be functionally deleted depending on how the antigen is presented to them. In particular, lack of a second signal to the T cells can induce tolerance

First/Second signals refers to the traditional view that T cell activation requires an antigen/MHC (first) signal followed by costimulatory interactions and/or cytokines (second signal). In this scheme, absence of the second signal can cause clonal anergy leading to tolerance.

High zone and Low zone tolerance. Tolerance is best induced by high levels of antigen (high zone), which tolerizes B cells. However some antigens in minute (low zone) doses (much less than would be immunogenic) can also tolerize the T cell populations.

Enhancement includes ways of inducing tolerance in transplantation surgery, where the graft survival is enhanced. The mechanism often involves interference with antigen presentation, for example by administration of anti-MHC class II antibody to block T cell mediated recognition of graft antigens, or by using anti-CD4 to interfere with immune recognition by the T cells.

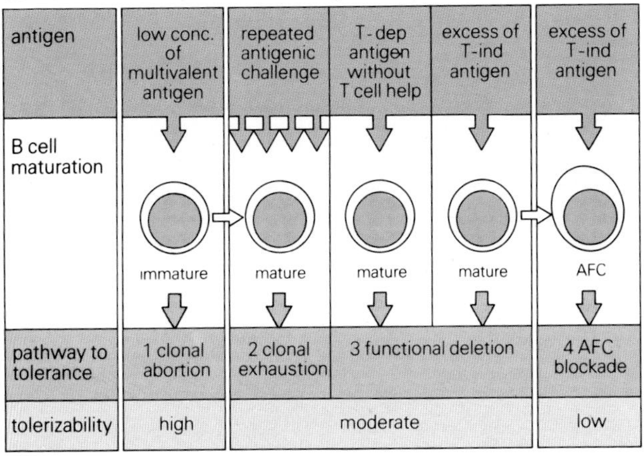

antigen	low conc. of multivalent antigen	repeated antigenic challenge	T-dep antigen without T cell help	excess of T-ind antigen	excess of T-ind antigen
B cell maturation	immature	mature	mature	mature	AFC
pathway to tolerance	1 clonal abortion	2 clonal exhaustion	3 functional deletion		4 AFC blockade
tolerizability	high	moderate			low

Fig. 3.23 Pathways to B cell tolerance.

Inflammation and Cell Migration | 4

INFLAMMATION

Inflammation is the response of tissues to injury, with the function of bringing serum molecules and cells of the immune system to the site of damage. The reaction consists of three components: 1) Increased blood supply to the region; 2) Increased capillary permeability in the affected area; 3) Emigration of cells out of the blood vessels and into the tissues. Inflammation is an ordered process, mediated by the appearance of intercellular adhesion molecules on endothelia and various inflammatory mediators released by tissue cells and leucocytes. Plasma enzyme systems are particularly important sources of inflammatory mediators. These include the complement, clotting, fibrinolytic (plasmin) and kinin systems. Also active are the mediators released by mast cells, basophils and platelets, as well as the eicosanoids generated by many cells at inflammatory sites. Generally, neutrophils are the first cells to appear at acute inflammatory sites, followed by macrophages and lymphocytes, if there is an immunological challenge.

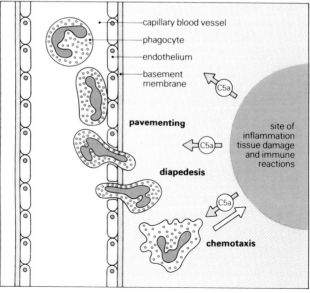

Fig. 4.1 Stages of chemotaxis.

Vasodilation is the dilation of the local blood vessels caused by the actions of mediators on the smooth muscle of the vessel wall, allowing increased blood flow.

Transudate/exudate. Normally only small molecules pass freely through the capillary wall. The fluid which passes through is a transudate. If inflammation occurs the endothelial cells are caused to retract, permitting large molecules to pass out as well. This fluid, which is also rich in cells, is an inflammatory exudate.

Adhesion and pavementing are the first stages of cell migration from the blood stream. Most leucocyte migration into inflammatory sites occurs across post-capillary venules. The cells first adhere to the endothelial cells. They then develop multi-point contacts, and flatten onto the endothelium. This process is called pavementing.

Diapedesis is the process by which cells migrate across the endothelium and into tissues. Adherent cells extend pseudopodia into the intercellular junctions between endothelial cells, before squeezing through the gap, dissolving the basement membrane and migrating out into the tissues.

Chemotaxis is directional movement of cells in response to an inflammatory mediator. Cells are highly sensitive to, and migrate up, concentration gradients of chemotactic molecules such as C5a, fMet,Leu,Phe (fMLP) and IL-8.

Chemokinesis is increased random (i.e. non-directional) movement of cells caused by inflammatory mediators (e.g. histamine).

Mediators of inflammation include the plasma enzyme systems, cells of the immune system and the pathogens themselves. The

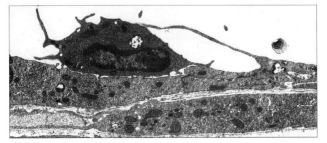

Fig. 4.2 Lymphocyte adhering to brain endothelium in encephalomyelitis. Courtesy of Dr Clive Hawkins.

mediator	origin	actions
histamine	mast cells basophils	increased vascular permeability smooth muscle contraction chemokinesis
5-hydroxy tryptamine (5HT)=serotonin	platelets mast cells (rodents)	increased vascular permeability smooth muscle contraction
platelet activating factor(PAF)	basophils neutrophils macrophages	mediator release from platelets increased vascular permeability smooth muscle contraction neutrophil activation
neutrophil chemotactic factor (NCF)	mast cells	neutrophil chemotaxis
IL-8	lymphocytes	monocyte localization
C3a	complement C3	mast cell degranulation smooth muscle contraction
C5a	complement C5	mast cell degranulation neutrophil and macrophage chemotaxis, neutrophil activation smooth muscle contraction increased capillary permeability
bradykinin	kinin system (kininogen)	vasodilation smooth muscle contraction increased vascular permeability pain
fibrinopeptides and fibrin break-down products	clotting system	increased vascular permeability neutrophil and macrophage chemotaxis
prostaglandin E2 (PGE2)	cyclooxygenase pathway	vasodilation potentiate increased vascular permeability produced by histamine and bradykinin
leukotriene B4 (LTB4)	lipoxygenase pathway	neutrophil chemotaxis synergises with PGE2 in increasing vascular permeability
leukotriene D4 (LTD4)	lipoxygenase pathway	smooth muscle contraction increased vascular permeability

Fig. 4.3 Mediators of acute inflammation.

principle mediators are listed opposite and the diagram below indicates how the various systems interact to generate them.

Kinins are generated following tissue injury. Bradykinin is generated by interactions of plasma enzyme systems by the action of kallikrein on high molecular weight kininogen. Lysyl bradykinin (kallidin) is generated by the action of tissue kallikrein on low molecular weight kininogen. They are exceptionally powerful vasoactive mediators.

Eicosanoids are mediators produced from arachidonic acid, which is released from membranes by the action of phospholipase A2. Arachidonic acid is converted into eicosanoids by mast cells and macrophages via two major pathways.

Prostaglandins (PG) and Thromboxanes (Tx) are produced by the action of cyclooxygenase on arachidonic acid. They have complex effects on the inflammatory response, often synergizing with other mediators.

Leukotrienes (LT) are produced by the lipoxygenase pathway which generates mediators of acute inflammation and the slow reacting substances important in hypersensitivity.

Formyl-methionyl peptides (fMet-) are bacterial products which are highly chemotactic for neutrophils.

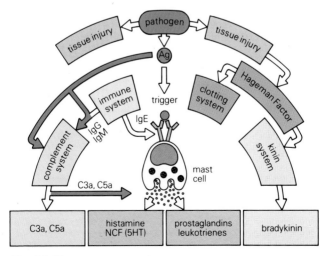

Fig. 4.4 Plasma enzyme systems.

COMPLEMENT

Complement is one of the serum enzyme systems. Its functions include mediating inflammation, opsonization of antigenic particles (including microorganisms) and causing membrane damage to pathogens. The system consists of serum molecules, which may be activated either via the 'classical' or 'alternative' pathways. Molecules of the classical pathway are designated C1, C2 etc. Alternative pathway molecules have letter designations, for example factor B (FB or just B). The properties of the components are given overleaf, and their receptors are on page 53

Enzyme cascade. The complement components interact with each other so that the products of one reaction form the enzyme for the next. Thus a small initial stimulus can trigger a cascade of activity. Small fragments of complement molecules produced by cleavage are subscripted (e.g. C3a,C5b). Inactivated enzymes are prefixed 'i' (e.g. iC3b), and active enzymes are indicated with a bar (e.g. $\overline{C3b,Bb}$).

The classical pathway (backshaded yellow) is activated by immune complexes binding to the C1q subcomponent of C1, which has six Fc binding sites. This induces enzymic cleavage of $\overline{C1r}$ and $\overline{C1s}$. C1s then splits C4a from C4 and C2b from C2 leaving $\overline{C4b,2a}$ which can then cleave C3.

The alternative pathway (properdin pathway or amplification loop) (backshaded purple) is activated in the presence of suitable surfaces or molecules, including microbial products. C3b can bind either H or B. Normally H is bound and C3b is inactivated by I, but in the presence of activators B is $\overline{bound\ and}$ then enzymically cleaved by D releasing Ba and leaving $\overline{C3b,Bb}$, an enzyme which can cleave C3. This gives a positive feedback (amplification) loop to generate more C3b.

C3 convertases including $\overline{C3b,Bb}$ and $\overline{C4b,2a}$, clip C3a from C3 to leave C3b. This has a labile binding site which allows it to covalently bind to nearby molecules with -OH or $-NH_2$ groups. C3b, together with a C3 convertase, can cleave C5.

The lytic pathway (backshaded orange) is activated when C5b is deposited on membranes. C5b associates C7, C8 and C9 to form the membrane attack complex.

Membrane attack complex (MAC) is a structure of C5b678 and polymeric C9 which traverses the target cell membrane and allows osmotic leakage from the cell.

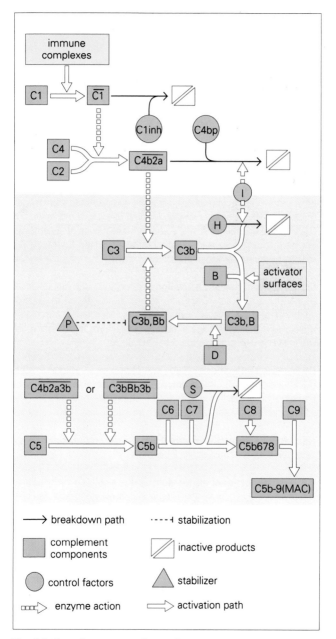

Fig. 4.5 Complement reaction pathways.

82

Complement fixation is the activation of complement followed by deposition of the activated components on immune complexes or cell membranes. C3b and C4b can bind covalently to nearby molecules via an internal thioester bond which becomes exposed on activation. The reactive group decays quickly by hydrolysis if a link is not formed. Hence complement is only deposited close to its site of activation.

Bystander lysis is the phenomenon where cells in close proximity to a site of complement activation have active components deposited on them and may then be lysed.

Anaphylatoxins C3a and C5a, cleaved from the N-termini of the α chains of C3 and C5, mediate inflammation by causing mast cell degranulation, smooth muscle contraction and increased capillary permeability. C5a is also chemotactic for neutrophils and monocytes. In this way these peptides mimic some of the reactions of anaphylaxis. They are substantially inactivated by removal of their C-terminal Arg residue by serum carboxypeptidases.

Control of complement activation is effected by the natural decay of the enzymically active convertases and the actions of the various inhibitors and inactivators listed opposite. Membrane associated molecules also alter the rate of complement breakdown. In- particular CR1, FH and DAF promote the decay of C3b,Bb.

Decay Accelerating Factor (DAF) and Membrane Cofactor Protein (MCP) are proteins normally present on many mammalian cell membranes which limit the activity of the alternative pathway and the development of C5 convertases.

Homologous Restriction Factor (HRF) is a membrane protein which limits the activity of autologous C8 and C9.

Paroxysmal nocturnal haemoglobinuria is a condition in which red cell breakdown occurs via the alternative pathway. Patients' red cells are deficient in control proteins (particularly DAF) and may also have low surface sialic acid.

Hereditary angioedema is a condition caused by a genetic deficiency of C1inh. There is uncontrolled local activation of C2 which undergoes conversion into a kinin which induces pathological local oedema.

Cobra Venom Factor (CVF) is cobra C3b, which forms a C3 convertase (CVF,Bb) which is not susceptible to inactivation by Fl. It can therefore be used to deplete mammalian C3.

component	mol. wt. (kD)	serum conc. (μg/ml)	no. of poly-peptides	function
C1q	410	150	18	form a Ca^{++}linked complex-Clq Clr$_2$ Cls$_2$; Clq binds to complexed Ig to activate the classical pathway
Clr	83	50	1	
Cls	83	50	1	
C4	210	550	3	classical pathway molecules, activated by Cls to form a C3 convertase, C4b2a
C2	115	25	1	
C3	180	1200	2	active C3 (C3b) opsonizes anything to which it binds and activates the lytic pathway. C3a causes mast cell degranulation and smooth muscle contraction. iC3b, C3d, C3e and C3g are breakdown products of C3b
C5	180	70	2	C5b on membranes initiates the lytic pathway. C5a is chemotactic for macrophages and neutrophils, causes smooth muscle contraction, mast cell degranulation and increased capillary permeability
C6	130	60	1	lytic pathway components which assemble in the presence of C5b to form the membrane attack complex and so may cause cell lysis
C7	120	50	1	
C8	155	55	3	
C9	75	60	1	
B	95	200	1	B binds to C3b in presence of alternative pathway activators,then is cleaved by D an active serum enzyme to form a C3 convertase C3b,Bb
D	25	10	1	
P (properdin)	185	25	4	stabilizes C3b,Bb to potentiate amplification loop activity
C4bp	550	250	7	C4bp binds C4b and H binds to C3b to act as cofactors for I which cleaves and inactivates C3b and C4b
H(β_1H)	150	500	1	
I(C3bina)	100	30	2	
Clinh	100	185	1	binds and inactivates Clr$_2$ and Cls$_2$
S-protein (vitro-nectin)	83	505	1	binds C5b-7, prevents attachment to membranes

Fig. 4.6 The complement components.

MECHANISMS OF CELL MIGRATION

Leucocyte migration is controlled by surface adhesion molecules which interact with complementary adhesion molecules expressed on vascular endothelium. Most leucocyte migration occurs across venules. Several patterns of cell migration can be distinguished, including: 1) Movement of lymphocytes into secondary lymphoid tissues; 2) Migration of neutrophils into tissues during an acute immune response, and migration of mononuclear cells into chronic inflammatory sites; 3) Migration of activated lymphocytes to inflammatory sites. Each pattern of migration is determined by particular sets of adhesion molecules. Following attachment to the endothelium pseudopodia probe the region around the interendothelial junction and extend towards the basement membrane. Enzymes released by the migrating cells dissolve the basement membrane and the cells move through the endothelium, disengaging their adhesion molecules. The cells may now acquire new adhesion molecules to allow them to interact with tissue cells and extracellular matrix components.

Adhesion molecules fall into several different structural groups. Some are constitutively expressed by cells (e.g. CR3 on mononuclear cells) whereas others may be induced by cytokines or cellular activation. Some adhesion molecules are retained in stores within the cell and may be quickly mobilized to the cell surface (e.g. LFA-1 present in neutrophil 'adhesomes', whereas others (e.g. ICAM-1 in endothelium) must be synthesized. The major groups of adhesion molecules are:

Integrins consist of an α and β chain both of which traverse the cell membrane. In general the α chain is unique to each molecule, whereas the β chain may be shared with other molecules in the family. Adhesion is magnesium dependent, and often depends on an Arg-Gly-Asp (RGD) sequence in the ligand molecule.

VLA (Very Late Antigens) is the designation of the β_1 integrin family, which includes two molecules which appear late on activated T cells and may be involved in binding to extracellular matrix.

Selectins (LECCAMS) include GMP-140, ELAM (endothelial leucocyte adhesion molecule) and MEL-14 (in mouse) or its human equivalent, the peripheral lymph node homing receptor. They each have a terminal lectin-like domain and are thought to bind to sugar residues on their target cell.

Intercellular adhesion molecules (ICAM-1, ICAM-2 and VCAM) belong to the immunoglobulin supergene family. ICAM-1 and ICAM-2 have homologous N-termini and bind to LFA-1.

CD44 (Pgp) is a widely distributed molecule also present on leuco-cytes and thought to be involved in transendothelial migration. Its structure suggests that it could interact with extracellular matrix.

Addressins are the proposed endothelial receptors which may confer tissue specificity on the migration pathways.

adhesion molecule	structure	location	ligand	function
GMP-140	selectin	endothelium neutrophils platelets	carbohydrate	acute inflammation neutrophil migration platelet adhesion
ELAM	selectin	endothelium	carbohydrate	neutrophil migration
ICAM-1	5 domains	endothelium leukocytes	LFA-1	enhances intercellular adhesion
ICAM-2	2 domains	endothelium	LFA-1	endothelial adhesion
VCAM	6 domains	endothelium	VLA-4	lymphocyte homing
Addressins	1 chain	endothelium	?	lymphocyte homing
MEL-14	selectin	lymphocytes	carbohydrate	binding to lymph node HEVs
VLA-1	integrin	lymphocytes	?	matrix binding
VLA-2	integrin	primed T cells	collagen	matrix binding
VLA-4	integrin	leucocytes	VCAM	endothelial binding
VLA-5	integrin	leucocytes	fibronectin	matrix binding
LFA-1	integrin	leucocytes	ICAM-2 ICAM-1	enhancing adhesion costimulatory signal
CR3	integrin	neutrophils macrophages	? & iC3b	neutrophil migration opsonization
CR4	integrin	macrophages	iC3b	opsonization

Fig. 4.7 Adhesion molecules.

Immunopathology | 5

IMMUNODEFICIENCY

Immunodeficiency is often identified in individuals by their increased susceptibility to infection, caused by a failure of one or more divisions of the immune system. Primary immunodeficiencies are inherited and may affect any part of the system. Examples include failure of lymphocyte development, impaired granulocyte functions, lack of macrophage receptors and absence of particular complement components. These deficiencies usually become apparent in the early months of life as immunity conferred by maternal antibodies wanes. Secondary, or acquired immunodeficiency is a consequence of many pathogenic infections, some of which directly attack the immune system (e.g. HIV infection) while others (e.g. malaria) subvert effective immune responses.

Severe Combined Immunodeficiency (SCID) is a group of conditions with leukopenia, impaired cell mediated immunity, low or absent antibody levels and undeveloped secondary lymphoid tissues. Some cases can be attributed to autosomal recessive adenosine deaminase deficiency or purine nucleoside phosphorylase deficiency. Other cases in which these enzymes are unaffected may

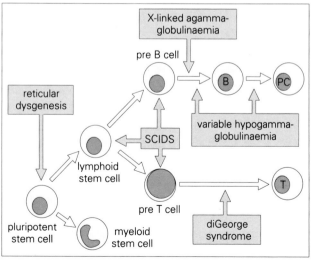

Fig. 5.1   Immunodeficiencies.

be X-linked or autosomal recessive traits, and one type may be related to inability to recombine antigen receptor molecules. The different forms of SCID may be correlated with the points on the lymphomyeloid differentiation pathways at which the deficiencies act.

DiGeorge Syndrome due to failed development of the third and fourth pharyngeal pouches results in thymic hypoplasia with low numbers of functionally active T cells. T cell numbers may rise to normal within 1 to 2 years.

X-linked agammaglobulinaemia (Bruton's disease). Patients with this condition have normal T cell functions and cell-mediated immunity to viral infections, but have very low immunoglobulin levels and cannot make antibody responses. Pre-B cells do not differentiate into mature B cells in this condition.

Variable hypogammaglobulinaemia is a variety of conditions with no clear pattern of inheritance, which affect B cell differentiation – B cells are often present, but do not develop into plasma cells. There is a relatively high incidence of autoimmunity and lymphoreticular neoplasias.

Ataxia telangiectasia, a neurological disease, also has an associated immunodeficiency. There is reduced T cell function and some Ig subclasses are deficient. It is thought to be related to an inability to repair DNA, and chromosomal breaks occur in the Ig genes.

Wiskott Aldrich syndrome has a severe associated immunodeficiency in which T cells make ineffective responses to antigens. Lymphocyte numbers are near normal, but antibody subclasses are abnormal and antibody is rapidly catabolized.

Thymoma, a thymocyte neoplasia, is associated with immunodeficiency and a number of autoimmune diseases, including myasthenia gravis and haemolytic anaemia.

Heavy chain disease is a B cell disorder, where cells produce incomplete Ig heavy chains.

Acquired Immune Deficiency Syndrome (AIDS) is due to infection with the retrovirus HIV-1. This can infect cells expressing CD4, including T helper cells and some APCs which also express low levels of CD4. $CD4^+$ T cell deficiency develops and this is associated with opportunistic infections and sometimes a fast growing form of Kaposi's sarcoma. B cells, Tc cells and phagocytes may be affected secondarily.

AUTOIMMUNE DISEASE

Autoantigens/autoantibodies refer to self molecules recognized as antigens and the antibodies which react against them.

Autoreactive cells are lymphocytes with receptors for autoantigens. These cells can potentially produce an autoimmune response, but do not necessarily do so.

Autoimmunity is the reaction of the immune system against the body's own tissues. To understand how autoimmune reactions can develop it is necessary to know the mechanisms by which self-tolerance is normally maintained. These include: 1) Sequestration of autoantigen in inaccessible sites; 2) Deletion of autoreactive T cells during thymic development; 3) Failure to process and present particular self molecules; 4) Induction of anergy in autoreactive T cells, due to lack of costimulatory signals and/or specific cytokines; 5) Suppressor cells and hormones (e.g. glucocorticoids). Failure of any of these mechanisms could lead to autoimmunity. For example, release of autoantigen following tissue damage circumvents (1), whereas provision of costimulatory signals to T cells which have recognized autoantigen circumvents (4).

T cell bypass. It is thought that self-tolerance is maintained at the T cell level - self-reactive T cells are deleted or anergized (Fig 5.2a). Autoreactive B cells may become activated by a mechanism which bypasses the tolerant T cells. For example, a cross-reactive exogenous antigen taken up by an autoreactive B cell could be presented to a T cell recognizing a non-self epitope, which then helps the B cell (Fig 5.2b). Alternatively, polyclonal stimulators such as EB virus (EBV) or LPS could stimulate the B cells directly (Fig 5.2c).

Autoregulatory failure. The control of some autoreactive cells is thought to be due to failure of appropriate antigen presentation or suppressor cells (Fig 5.2d). If there is a failure of suppression or if the autoantigen is presented in an immunogenic fashion then autoimmunity may develop (Fig 5.2e).

Autoimmune diseases occur when autoimmune reactions result in pathological tissue damage. In general they are either organ-specific or organ non-specific.

Organ-specific autoimmune diseases are directed primarily at particular tissues, e.g. anti-thyroglobulin in Hashimoto's thyroiditis or to pancreatic β cells in diabetes. Organ-specific autoantibodies tend to occur together in particular individuals and their relatives.

Organ non-specific autoimmune diseases are directed to widely distributed autoantigens such as the anti-DNA antibody in systemic lupus erythematosus. These conditions often produce type III immune complex mediated hypersensitivity reactions.

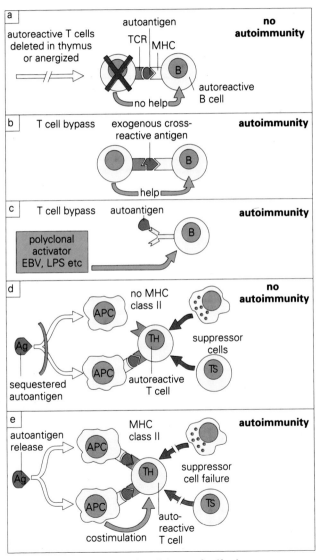

Fig. 5.2 Maintenance and breakdown of self tolerance.

HYPERSENSITIVITY

Hypersensitivity describes an immune response which occurs in an exaggerated or inappropriate form. In some cases responses may occur against inoccuous external antigens, such as pollen in hayfever. In other cases responses against genuine pathogens are generated which are out of proportion to the damage caused by the pathogen. Also of great importance are the different kinds of tissue damage seen in autoimmune diseases: these are in effect hypersensitivity reactions, since any response to a self-antigen is 'inappropriate'. The hypersensitivity reactions were classified by Gell and Coombs, according to the speed of the reaction and the immune mechanisms involved. Although they are classified sepa-

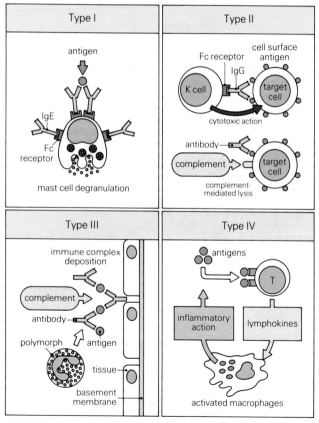

Fig. 5.3   Four types of hypersensitivity reaction.

rately, in practice they do not necessarily occur in isolation from each other. Moreover, several different immune reactions may be subsumed in a single type.

Type I (Immediate) hypersensitivity is seen in allergic asthma, hayfever and some types of excema. It develops within minutes of exposure to antigen and is dependent on the activation of mast cells and the release of mediators of acute inflammation. Mast cells bind IgE via their surface Fcε receptors and when antigen crosslinks the IgE, the mast cells degranulate releasing vasoactive amines which produce acute inflammation. Prostaglandins and leukotrienes, produced by arachidonic acid metabolism, contribute to a delayed component of the reaction which often develops hours after the original exposure to antigen.

Type II (Antibody-mediated) hypersensitivity is caused by antibody to cell surface antigens and components of the extracellular matrix. These antibodies can sensitize the cells for antibody-dependent cytotoxic attack by K cells or for complement mediated lysis. Type II hypersensitivity is seen in the destruction of red cells in transfusion reactions and in haemolytic disease of the newborn. Tissue destruction in autoimmune diseases, such as myasthenia gravis and Goodpasture's syndrome is also partly antibody-mediated.

Type III (Immune complex mediated) hypersensitivity is caused by the deposition of antigen/antibody complexes in tissue and blood vessels. This tends to occur particularly at sites of filtration such as the glomerulus. The complexes activate complement and attract polymorphs and macrophages to the site. These cells may exocytose their granule contents and release reactive oxygen intermediates (ROIs) to cause local tissue damage. The antigens in the complexes may come from persistent pathogenic infections (e.g. malaria), from inhaled antigens (e.g. extrinsic allergic alveolitis) or from the host's own tissue, in autoimmune disease. These conditions are all characterized by a high antigen load, which may be associated with a weak or ineffective antibody response.

Type IV (Delayed) hypersensitivity arises more than 24 hours after encounter with the antigen and is mediated by antigen sensitized CD4$^+$ T cells which release cytokines, attracting macrophages to the site and activating them. The macrophages produce tissue damage which may develop into chronic granulomatous reactions if the antigen persists. This type of hypersensitivity is seen in skin contact reactions and in the response to some chronic pathogens, such as *Mycobacterium leprae*, *M. tuberculosis* and *Schistosoma* spp.

92

TYPE I (IMMEDIATE) HYPERSENSITIVITY

Allergy originally meaning altered reactivity on a second contact with an antigen, now means type I hypersensitivity.

Allergen is any antigen which induces a type I reaction.

Sensitization in this context is the process by which a susceptible individual develops an allergen-specific IgE response. The IgE may bind to the high affinity FcεR on mast cells, thereby sensitizing them for triggering by the allergen.

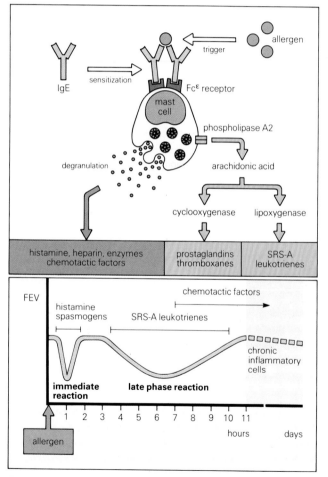

Fig. 5.4 Type I hypersensitivity.

Triggering of mast cells occurs when antigen crosslinks the cell surface IgE, causing an influx of Ca^{++}, resulting in degranulation and activation of phospholipase A2. Mast cells can also be directly triggered by anaphylatoxins, C3a and C5a.

Phospholipase A2 is a membrane-associated enzyme which releases arachidonic acid, the initial substrate for the lipoxygenase pathway with produces leukotrienes, and the cyclooxygenase pathway which produces prostaglandins and thromboxanes.

Atopy describes conditions which manifest type I hypersensitivity, including asthma, hayfever and excema. These tend to cluster in families. These reactions are exemplified opposite by allergic asthma induced by breathing an allergen.

Immediate and Late phase reactions. Following bronchial provocation with an allergen there is an immediate reduction in airway patency measured as a fall in forced expiratory volume (FEV), caused by histamine, prostaglandins and via the action of PAF on platelets. After several hours a late phase reaction develops caused primarily by leukotrienes and cytokines. Inflammatory cells, including macrophages, basophils and other polymorphs arrive under chemotactic influences. Analagous immediate and late reactions occur in allergic skin reactions.

SRS-A (Slow Reacting Substance-A) a mediator of the late phase reaction consists primarily of leukotrienes C4 and D4.

Anaphylaxis is a systemic type I reaction seen in sensitized animals injected with allergen. The release of vasoactive amines and spasmogens causes smooth muscle contraction, increased vascular permeability and a fall in blood pressure. Respiratory or circulatory failure may ensue.

Passive Cutaneous Anaphylaxis (PCA) is an assay for antigen-specific IgE in which an animal is sensitized by subcutaneous injection of test serum and then challenged with allergen. If specific IgE is present in the serum, the local mast cells degranulate, causing increased local vascular permeability.

Prausnitz Kustner reaction is the equivalent to PCA performed in man. The positive reaction gives a wheal at the injection site.

Prick test is used to determine an individual's (type I) sensitivity to allergens, which are pricked onto the skin. Sensitive individuals generate a wheal and flare reaction.

TYPE II (ANTIBODY MEDIATED) HYPERSENSITIVITY

Type II hypersensitivity is caused by antibody directed to membranes and cell surface antigens. Complement may be activated and effector cells with Fcγ receptors and C3 receptors can then engage the target tissue. Membrane attack complexes may also be formed, to potentiate the damage. The site of damage depends on the antibodies involved.

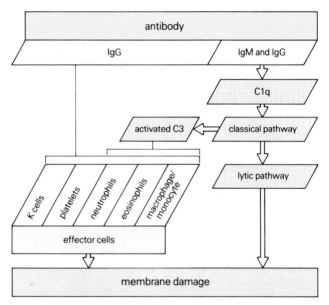

Fig. 5.5 Type II hypersensitivity.

Transfusion reactions occur when mismatched donor blood is infused into a recipient. The recipient may have naturally occurring antibodies to the foreign cells, as happens with the ABO blood group system, or they may develop after infusion. The antibodies can cause complement-dependent lysis or sequestration of the sensitized cells in spleen and liver.

Blood groups are systems of allotypically variable erythrocyte surface antigens, some of which occur on other tissues also. The more common ones are listed in Figure 5.6.

Chido and Rogers blood group antigens are the electrophoretically slow and fast allotypes respectively of human C4, which have adsorbed to the red cell surface.

Haemolytic Disease of the Newborn (HDNB) is caused by maternal antibodies to foetal red cells, which cross the placenta and destroy them. The mother becomes sensitized by foetal red cells entering her circulation at birth, so that the first child is usually unaffected. The most common cases involve Rhesus-negative mothers carrying Rhesus-positive children.

Rhesus prophylaxis is the administration of anti-Rhesus D antibody to Rhesus-negative mothers immediately after delivering a Rhesus-positive child in order to destroy the Rh^+ cells and thus prevent them sensitizing the mother.

Autoimmune haemolytic anaemia is caused by autoantibodies to red cells producing cell destruction by lysis or sequestration. The antibodies may be either 'warm agglutinins' or 'cold agglutinins' depending on the temperature at which they bind.

Myasthenia Gravis (MG) is a disease with muscle weaknesss, caused by impaired neuromuscular transmission, partly caused by autoantibodies to acetylcholine receptors.

Goodpastures syndrome has a type II reaction in which autoantibodies damage lung and kidney basement membranes.

system	gene loci	antigens	phenotype frequencies	
ABO	1	A, B or O	A B AB O	42% 8% 3% 47%
Rhesus	3 closely linked loci: major antigen=RhD	C or c D or d E or e	RhD^+ RhD^-	85% 15%
Kell	1	K or k	K k	9% 91%
Duffy	1	Fy^a, Fy^b or Fy	$Fy^a Fy^b$ Fy^a Fy^b Fy	46% 20% 34% 0.1%
MN	1	M or N	MM NN MN	28% 50% 22%

Fig. 5.6 **Five major human blood group systems.**

TYPE III (IMMUNE COMPLEX MEDIATED) HYPERSENSITIVITY

Immune complexes are combinations of antigen and antibody, often with associated complement components.

Immune complex deposition. Type III hypersensitivity results from the deposition of immune complexes in blood vessel walls and tissues. Complexes can activate platelets (in man) and basophils via Fc receptors to release vasoactive amines which cause endothelial cell retraction and increased vascular permeability leading to complex deposition. Complexes also activate complement, releasing C3a and C5a both of which activate basophils, while C5a is chemotactic for neutrophils. Phagocytes which are unable to endocytose the deposited complexes, release granule contents and ROIs causing local tissue damage. Complexes tend to deposit at sites of high pressure, filtration or turbulence, particularly the kidney.

Immune complex clearance. In man circulating complexes are normally taken up by erythrocytes and carried to the liver where they are transferred to, and degraded by phagocytes. Factors which affect

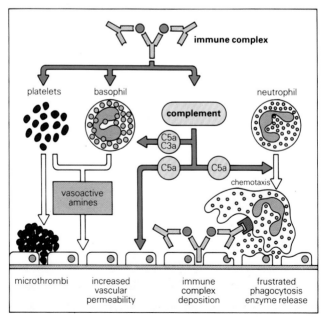

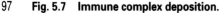

Fig. 5.7   Immune complex deposition.

clearance include: a) size of the complexes; b) class and affinity of the antibody; c) valency of the antigen; and d) the amount of complex. This last factor explains why immune complex disease occurs in infections which release large amounts of antigen, and in autoimmune diseases where there is a ready supply of autoantigen.

Immune complex diseases result when excessive immune complex deposition occurs in particular organs.

Serum sickness is a type III reaction which occurs in individuals injected with foreign serum. Antibodies are made to the serum antigens and there is massive immune complex formation, producing arthritis and nephritis.

Arthus reaction is a skin reaction seen as an area of redness and swelling which is maximal 5–6 hours after intradermal injection of antigen. It is caused by IgG binding to the injected antigen and triggering inflammation by type III mechanisms.

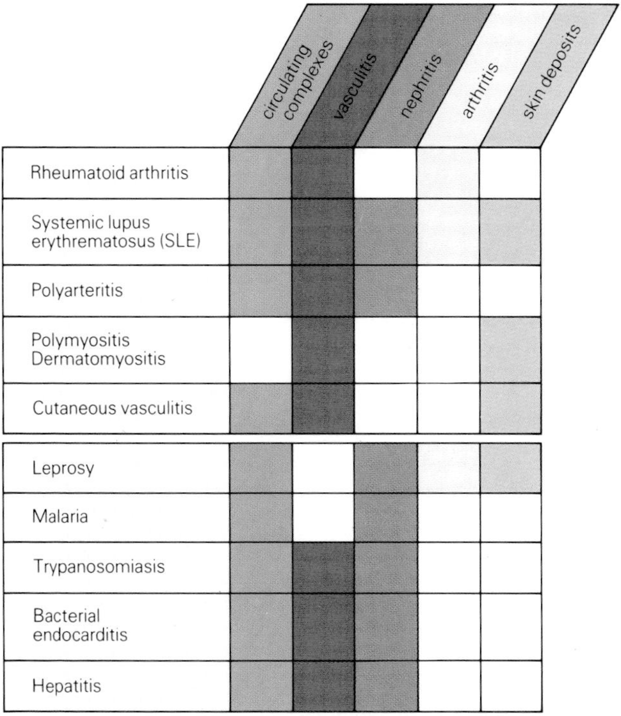

	circulating complexes	vasculitis	nephritis	arthritis	skin deposits
Rheumatoid arthritis	●	●		●	
Systemic lupus erythrematosus (SLE)	●	●	●	●	●
Polyarteritis	●	●	●		
Polymyositis Dermatomyositis		●			●
Cutaneous vasculitis	●	●			
Leprosy	●		●	●	
Malaria	●		●		
Trypanosomiasis	●	●	●		
Bacterial endocarditis	●	●	●		
Hepatitis	●	●	●		

Fig. 5.8 Immune complex diseases: sites of deposition.

TYPE IV (DELAYED) HYPERSENSITIVITY (DTH)

This includes a number of reactions which are maximal at more than 12 hours after challenge with antigen, and which are dependent on antigen-reactive T cells, rather than antibody. The cells responsible are a functionally defined subgroup of $CD4^+$ T_H cells sometimes referred to as T_D cells. At least four types of reaction have been described, but they may occur concommitantly or sequentially in the reaction to a particular antigen. For example, if an antigenic stimulus persists a tuberculin-type reaction may develop into a granuloma.

Jones Mote reactions (Cutaneous basophil hypersensitivity) appear within 24 hours of skin challenge with antigen. The area beneath the epidermis becomes infiltrated with basophils over 1 - 6 days with maximal skin swelling on day 1. The response is thought to be normally regulated by suppressor cells.

Contact hypersensitivity produces an excematous skin reaction in sensitized human which is maximal 48 hours after contact with the allergen. The allergens may be large molecules or small haptens

type	Jones-Mote	contact	tuberculin	granulomatous
reaction time	24 hours	48 hours	48 hours	4 weeks
clinical appearance	skin swelling	eczema	local induration and swelling ± fever	skin induration
histological appearance	basophils, lymphocytes, mononuclear cells	mononuclear cells, oedema, raised epidermis	mononuclear cells, lymphocytes and monocytes, reduced macrophages	epithelioid cell granuloma, giant cells, macrophages, fibrosis, ± necrosis
antigen	intradermal antigen eg. ovalbumin	epidermal: eg. nickel, rubber, poison ivy etc.	dermal: tuberculin, mycobacterial and leishmanial antigens	persistent Ag or Ag/Ab complexes in macrophages or 'non immunological' eg. talcum powder

Fig. 5.9   Summary of the important characteristics of four types of delayed hypersensitivity reaction.

(e.g. nickel) which attach to normal body proteins, and modify them. Langerhans cells pick up these antigens and present them to T cells in local lymph nodes. Reactions are characterized by mononuclear cell infiltration with oedema and microvesicle formation in the epidermis. The dermis is usually infiltrated by an increased number of leucocytes.

Tuberculin-type hypersensitivity was originally a reaction produced by subcutaneous injection of tuberculin in patients with tuberculosis who responded with fever and swelling at the injection site. The term usually refers to the skin reaction induced by antigen which is maximal at 48 hours after challenge and consists of lymphocytes and mononuclear phagocytes. If the antigenic stimulus persists a granulomatous reaction may develop. This type of reaction may be induced in a sensitized subject by several microbial and non-microbial antigens.

Granulomatous reactions develop where there is a persistent stimulus which macrophages cannot eliminate. Non-antigenic particles (e.g. talc) induce non-immunological granulomas while persistent pathogens, such as *Mycobacteria* spp. and *Schistosomula* spp induce immunological granulomas. The lesion consists of a palisade of epithelioid cells and macrophages surrounding the infectious agent which is in turn surrounded by a cuff of lymphocytes. Collagenous capsules may also develop around some pathogens due to fibroblast proliferation.

Epithelioid cells, large flattened cells with large amounts of endoplasmic reticulum are seen in granulomas and are thought to be derived from macrophages, although they have fewer phagosomes than macrophages

Giant cells are large multi-nucleated cells present in granulomas, which are thought to be derived from the fusion of macrophages and/or epithelioid cells.

Migration Inhibition Test (MIT) This assay detects sensitized T cells. Test cells are packed with monocytes and antigen in capillary tubes and then cultured on agar plates. If antigen-sensitive T cells are present they release cytokines (MIF, IL-8 etc.) which limit the migration of the monocytes.

Patch test is used to assess type IV contact hypersensitivity to allergens. The allergen is applied to the skin and the development of an excematous reaction 48 hours later indicates that the subject is sensitive.

100

ANIMAL MODELS AND MUTANT STRAINS

Different strains of animals with impaired immune systems have been particularly useful in modelling human immunodeficiencies and autoimmune diseases. It must be emphasized that the resemblance may only be in the appearance of the diseases. In some cases (e.g. nude strains) the defect is determined by a single gene locus, but autoimmunity in the autoimmune strains depends on multiple genetic loci which interact with each other. Figure 5.10 lists some of the more important strains.

Genotype/Phenotype. The genotype is the genetic composition of an animal, whereas its phenotype is the observed characteristics which depend on how the genes are expressed.

Haplotype is a set of genes located on a single chromosome, and the characteristics dependent on them. In outbred populations the maternal and paternal chromosomes usually differ, so an individual has two haplotypes of each set of genes.

Inbred strains of animals are made by repeated brother x sister matings in successive generations giving a strain with identical sets of autosomes. If by chance a pair of identical chromosomes occurs in the F_1 animals, inbreeding ensures that the pair remains fixed in the genome of subsequent generations. By repeated inbreeding, all the chromosome pairs become (and will remain) homozygous. Strains homozygous at the MHC loci have been essential in the examination of the role of this locus in graft rejection and antigen presentation.

Recombinant strains are produced by crossing different inbred strains. On rare occasions, crossing over occurs in the F_1 animal so that the affected chromosome has different haplotypes at each end. These strains are used to identify the segment of chromosome responsible for a particular characteristic.

Recombinant inbred strains are produced by crossing strains (a x b) and then inbreeding from the offspring. This gives strains which have identical sets of chromosomes, but each set will either be of the a type or b type at random. They are used to determine which chromosomes carry the genes for each trait.

Congenic strains are bred to be identical to each other except at some chosen locus. For example, an $H-2^k$ congenic animal would have the MHC locus of the k haplotype superimposed on a background of genes from a non-$H-2^k$ strain

bm mutants are strains of mice derived from an H-2^b strain and which developed mutations in the H-2 region (mostly H-2K). Mice with these mutations, designated H-2^{bm}, induce graft rejection reactions in H-2^b mice.

strain/species	characteristics
nude mouse nude rat	The nude mutant (nu) lacks a thymus and all T cells. A linked locus produces hairlessness
beige mouse	The beige mutant (bg) has several defects including lack of NK cells
NZB mouse	Autoimmunity including haemolytic anaemia with failure of immunoregulation
(NZB/NZW) F$_1$ mouse	Autoimmunity includung immune complex nephritis - possible model of systemic lupus erythematosus
MRL. lpr	Autoimmunity. The lpr gene produces T cell lymphoproliferation - model of rheumatoid arthritis
NOD mouse (non-obese diabetic)	Autoimmune reaction to pancreatic β cells - model of type II insulin-dependent diabetes
BXSB	Autoimmune lupus - like syndrome with B cell lymphoproliferation
SCID mouse	Aberrant lymphocyte differentiation model of SCID in man
CBA/n	Lacks a B cell subset (lyb5). Fails to respond to some T-independent antigens
C3H/HeJ	B cells lack a receptor for LPS
DBA/2Ha	X-linked defect. B cells lack a receptor for T cell Replacing Factor (TRF)
B/B rat	Spontaneous autoimmune diabetes and thyroid autoimmunity
buffalo rat	A proportion develop autoimmune thyroiditis and/or destruction of pancreatic β cell
obese chicken	Autoimmune thyroiditis - model of Hashimoto's disease

Fig. 5.10 Characteristics of some immunologically aberrant experimental strains.

MHC TYPING

Polymorphism refers to the numbers of variants seen in different individuals at the same gene locus. MHC loci are highly polymorphic. These variants may be detected at the level of the gene, by RFLP analysis or direct sequencing, or they may be detected in the expressed MHC molecules by the techniques of tissue typing.

Tissue typing is the technique used to determine the MHC specificities carried on an individual's cells. There are two main ways of doing this, either serologically or by MLC. Since MHC molecules occur on the cell surface they can be recognized as antigens by allogeneically different individuals and antisera can be raised to them. Typing is performed by adding antisera of defined specificity (e.g. anti-HLA-B8) to the cell to be typed (usually lymphocytes). Addition of complement kills the cells and this can be visualized by staining with trypan blue which is taken up by dead cells (Fig 5.11 right).

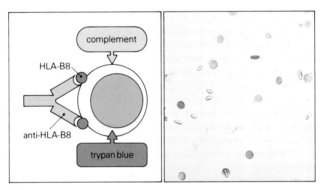

Fig. 5.11 Tissue typing – serological.

Typing sera, specific for particular MHC molecules were originally made by immunizing allogeneic individuals with cells and absorbing out unwanted specificities. Monoclonal antibodies to all determinants are now available.

Public (supratypic) and Private specificities. Antibodies raised against framework parts of MHC molecules often cross-react with several MHC antigens; these recognize public specificities, whereas antibodies which bind to only one MHC molecule are said to recognize private specificities.

Mixed Lymphocyte Culture/Reaction (MLC/MLR) is a technique for typing cells, in which lymphocytes of different individuals are cocultured. If the cells differ they are stimulated to divide. The test can be performed either with each set of cells reacting to the other (two way MLR), or with one set (stimulator) treated so that it cannot respond and only the proliferation of the responding (test) cells is measured (one way MLR). In the example shown below, the test cells Dw3,7 reacts to the stimulator (typing) cell Dw4,4, but the test cell Dw4,7 shares a haplotype with the typing cell and does not respond. Lack of response indicates therefore that the test cell and typing cell share a specificity.

Homozygous typing cells are cells with two identical MHC haplotypes. Human typing cells often come from the offspring of first cousin marriages.

Lymphocyte activating determinants (Lads) are the cell surface determinants which induce an MLR. MHC class II molecules are primarily responsible.

Primed Lymphocyte Test (PLT). This is a highly sensitive MLC assay for detecting Lads, in which the test cells are mixed with lymphocytes previously primed to a particular Lad by homozygous typing cells. The primed cells proliferate rapidly if the test cell carries the Lad of the original homozygous priming cell - primed cells, *not* the test cells, proliferate.

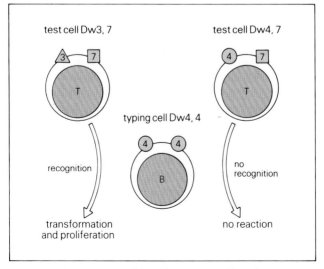

Fig. 5.12 Tissue typing – Mixed Lymphocyte Reaction.

HLA ALLOANTIGEN SPECIFICITIES

Numerous genetic variants have been identified at all the class I and class II loci, by sequencing the genome. Only a proportion of these variants can be identified by tissue typing techniques, since not all can induce alloantibodies, or be recognized by MLR. The full nomenclature for an MHC haplotype gives its gene designation, which includes a description of the specificities associated with it. For example, variant DRB1*0406 is present in the HLA-DR locus and affects the B1 gene encoding the first of the DR-β chains in this haplotype. It produces a molecule which expresses the DR4 specificity (04..) and is the sixth variant of this type identified so far (..06). Figure 5.13 gives the variants identifiable by tissue typing. Numbers in brackets are previous designations, now subdivided.

Class I Loci			Class II Loci		
HLA-A	HLA-B	HLA-C	HLA-DP	HLA-DQ	HLA-DR
A1	B7	Cw1	DPw1	DQw5 (w1)	DR1
A2	B8	Cw2	DPw2	DQw6 (w1)	DR'BR'
A3	B13	Cw3	DPw3	DQw2	DRw15(2)
All	B14	Cw5	DPw4	DQw7 (w3)	DRw16 (2)
A24 (9)	Bw65 (14)	Cw6	DPw5	DQw8 (w3)	DRw17 (3)
A25 (10)	Bw62 (15)	Cw7	DPw6	DQw9 (w3)	DRw18 (3)
A26 (10)	B18	Cw11	DP'Cp63'	DQw4	DR4
A29 (w19)	B27				DRw11 (5)
A30 (w19)	B35				DRw12 (5)
A31 (w19)	B37				DRw13 (w6)
A32 (w19)	B38 (16)				DRw14 (w6)
A33 (w19)	B39 (16)				DR7
Aw 68 (28)	Bw60 (40)				DRw8
Aw 69 (28)	B40				DR9
	Bw41				DRw10
	Bw42				DRw52a
	B44 (12)				DRw52b
	Bw46				DRw53
	Bw47				DRw15 (2)
	B49 (21)				DRw16 (2)
	B51 (5)				
	Bw52 (5)				
	Bw57 (17)				
	Bw58 (17)				

Fig. 5.13 HLA variants identified by tissue typing.

TRANSPLANTATION

Tissue transplants and immune reactions between cells of different individuals can be divided according to the donor/recipient combination, as follows:

Xenogeneic/xenografts describe immune reactions or tissue grafting between different species,
Allogeneic/allografts are reactions or grafting between genetically non-identical members of the same species,
Syngeneic/isografts are between genetically identical individuals,
Autografts are made with the recipient's own tissues.

Laws of transplantation state that grafts will be accepted if the recipient shares histocompatibility genes with the graft donor. So, in the examples below, a strain A mouse accepts a strain A graft but not a strain B graft. The (AxB)F1 mouse accepts the B graft because it has B genes, but the B mouse rejects the (AxB)F1 graft because it lacks the A genes.

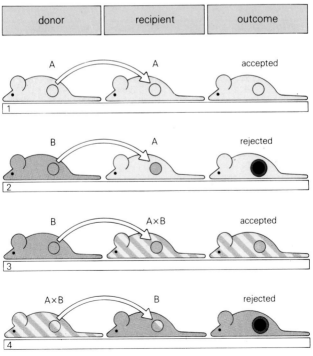

Fig. 5.14 The laws of transplantation.

Histocompatibility concerns the ability of an individual to accept grafts from another individual.

Histocompatibility genes determine whether a graft is accepted. A large number of gene loci affect rejection, but the MHC is most important. Although the MHC was first identified for its role in graft rejection this is not its physiological function.

Minor histocompatibility loci encode allelically variable molecules which induce weak graft rejection. There are up to 30 such loci in the mouse, H–1, H–3 etc. (H–2 is the mouse MHC). In man, even in MHC matched transplants (e.g. between siblings), graft rejection reactions can still occur, presumably due to minor locus differences. Reactions induced by these antigens can usually be suppressed, whereas MHC-induced reactions cannot.

H-Y is a monomorphic histocompatibility antigen encoded on the male (Y) chromosome. When female mice receive grafts from males of the same strain they sometimes recognize the H-Y antigen and reject the graft, whereas males accept grafts from females.

Transplantation antigens are allogeneic cell surface molecules recognized by T cells. MHC molecules are particularly important in inducing rejection. It appears that rejection due to minor loci differences is often due to the presentation of allelically variant molecules by the graft MHC molecules.

First and Second set rejection. The immune reactions which produce graft rejection display specificity and memory. For example, a

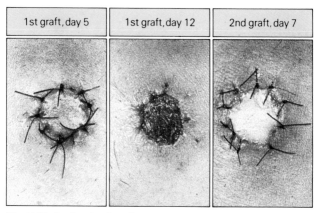

1st graft, day 5	1st graft, day 12	2nd graft, day 7

Fig. 5.15 Graft rejection displays immunological memory.

skin allograft in man will normally be rejected in 10 – 14 days (first set) but if a second allograft from the same individual (or one with the same tissue type) is given, the recipient will reject it more rapidly, usually in 5 – 7 days (second set).

Rejection reactions are induced by recipient TH cells which recognize allogeneic MHC molecules. These can activate graft infiltrating mononuclear cells to damage the graft. Alternatively Tc cells recognizing allogeneic class I MHC molecules can kill them, just as they kill infected cells.

Passenger cells are donor leucocytes present in graft tissue. They are thought to be particularly important in sensitizing TH cells to donor antigens, since they express class II MHC molecules and can migrate into the host lymphatic system.

Crossmatching. To avoid graft rejection the tissue type of the donor and recipient are crossmatched. All donor/recipients are matched for the ABO blood group, and where practical, for as many class I and II specificities as possible. The greater the number of shared specificities (particularly class II matches), the higher the chance of graft survival.

Privileged tissues. Some allogeneic graft tissues induce only weak immune reactions, e.g. liver. One explanation is that the privileged tissues express relatively few MHC antigens.

Privileged sites are areas where implanted grafts are largely isolated from the immune system, e.g. the cornea lacks a lymphatic drainage, and corneal allografts often fail to sensitize the recipient.

Hyperacute/Acute/Chronic rejection describe the speed of rejection in organs such as kidney. Hyperacute reactions occur within minutes of implantation and are caused by preformed antibody to the graft. Acute rejection occurs within two weeks of grafting, due to prior senzitisation of the recipient to histocompatibility antigens. Chronic rejection develops later due to the development of sensitivity to graft antigens. This sometimes occurs after the cessation of immunosuppression necessitated by infection.

Graft versus Host Disease (GvHD) is a condition where immunocompetent donor cells (e.g. from a bone marrow graft) recognize and react against the recipient's tissues, either because the recipient is immunosuppressed or cannot recognize the allogeneic cells. Sensitized donor TH cells can recruit macrophages to cause pathological damage especially in skin, gut epithelium and liver.

MHC DISEASE ASSOCIATIONS

Virtually every disease involving immune reactions, is preferentially associated with particular haplotypes of MHC molecules. For example, individuals with the class I molecule HLA-B27 are 90 times more likely to develop ankylosing spondylitis than people lacking this allele. The table opposite lists some of the diseases which show strong associations with particular MHC haplotypes. These disease associations are due to two factors that are central to the workings of the immune system: 1) MHC molecules are highly polymorphic, i.e. varying between loci and between individuals; and 2) MHC molecules are central to all aspects of antigen presentation. The corollary is that different MHC molecules may be better or worse at presenting different antigen peptides to T cells - some haplotypes permit strong immune responses, whereas others only allow weak ones. Indeed MHC class II molecules were first identified as immune response (Ir) genes. It follows, that since MHC genes control the ability to make immune responses, they also partly control disease susceptibility, in any condition where immune reactions occur.

Relative risk is the risk of developing a disease when a particular HLA haplotype is present compared to when it is absent. A relative risk of greater than one indicates that the haplotype is more prevalent in patients than in normal individuals, whereas a relative risk of less than one indicates a protective effect.

Linkage occurs between sets of genes on a single chromosome, such as the HLA complex. Unless crossover between maternal and paternal chromosomes occurs, a linked gene complex will be inherited as a block. Some diseases such as narcolepsy show strong MHC associations, although they appear to have no immunological component. The particular MHC haplotypes are probably linked to the real disease susceptibility gene(s).

Linkage disequilibrium refers to the finding that some pairs of genes are found together more frequently than would be expected by chance, that is more than the product of their individual gene frequencies. There are two possible explanations for this: 1) There is a selective advantage in inheriting the entire block of genes; or 2) Two genes have appeared together by chance, and there has been insufficient evolutionary time to separate them. Many sets of MHC molecules are linked, e.g. HLA-A1 with HLA-B8 and HLA-A3 with HLA-B7. Consequently, if one MHC molecule is associated with a disease, then any linked haplotypes will also be associated with the disease, although they do not necessarily contribute to the disease association.

disease	haplotypes	relative risk*
Rheumatoid arthritis	DR4	5.8
	DR3	5.0
	DR3 & DR4	14.0
Juvenile rheumatoid arthritis	B27	4.5
Ankylosing spondylitis	B27	90.0
Reiter's disease	B27	33.0
Post-shigella arthritis	B27	20.7
Post-salmonella arthritis	B27	17.6
Graves disease	DR3	3.5
	B35	5.0
Hashimoto's thyroiditis	DR3	2.6
Insulin dependent diabetes	DR3	5.7
Addison's disease	DR3	8.8
Multiple sclerosis	DR2	3.8
Myasthenia gravis	B8	3.4
	DR3	3.0
Psoriasis vulgaris	B37	6.4
	B13	4.7
	B17	4.7
	Cw6	13.3
Dermatitis herpitiformis	B8	8.7
	DR3	56.4
Goodpastures syndrome	DR2	13.1
Chronic active hepatitis	B8	9.0
	DR3	13.9
Coeliac disease	B8	8.3
	Dw3	10.9
Haemochromatosis	A3	8.2
	B14	4.7

Fig. 5.16 MHC Disease Associations (European caucasoids).
*Precise values vary between studies.

Immunological Tests and Techniques | 6

ASSAYS FOR ANTIGEN AND ANTIBODY

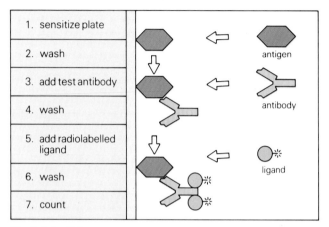

1. sensitize plate	
2. wash	
3. add test antibody	
4. wash	
5. add radiolabelled ligand	
6. wash	
7. count	

Fig. 6.1 Radioimmunoassay.

Radioimmunoassay (RIA) includes a variety of techniques which use radiolabelled reagents to detect antigen or antibody. Antibody may be detected using plates sensitized with antigen. Test antibody is applied and this is detected by the addition of a radiolabelled ligand specific for that antibody. The amount of ligand bound to the plate is proportional to the amount of test antibody.

Ligands/Conjugates are made by covalently coupling two molecules together. RIA ligands are usually antibody molecules or protein A, covalently bound to ^{125}I.

Protein A and Protein G are cell wall components of staphylococci which bind specifically to IgG (Fc) of most species at a site between Cγ2 and Cγ3.

Radioallergosorbent Test (RAST) is specialized form of RIA for detecting antigen-specific IgE, in which antigen is covalently coupled to cellulose discs. Antigen-specific IgE binding to the disc is detected using radiolabelled anti-IgE.

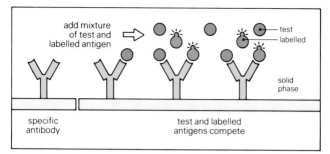

Fig. 6.2 Competition radioimmunoassay.

Competition radioimmunoassay is the classical RIA. It is used to detect antigens. Specific antibody is bound to a solid phase, and a mixture of test (unlabelled) and labelled antigen is applied. Labelled and unlabelled antigens compete with each other for the antibodies' binding sites. The greater the amount of test antigen that is present, the less labelled antigen will bind to the antibody. Calibration curves using known quantities of unlabelled antigen are established. The technique is often used for assaying hormones.

Radioimmunosorbent Test (RIST) is a competition RIA test as used to detect IgE (the antigen), in which test IgE is competed with labelled IgE on plates sensitized with anti-IgE.

Capture radioimmunoassays use antigen or antibody bound to the solid phase to capture molecules from the test solution, which are then detected with radiolabelled reagents. For example, solid phase anti-IgM captures IgM from the test solution, and the antigen-specific IgM is detected with a labelled antigen. The assay can be modified to detect antigen captured on solid phase IgG and identified with labelled IgG.

Sandwich radioimmunoassays are used to detect antibodies in systems where the test antibody acts as a bridge between solid phase unlabelled antigen and labelled antigen. Labelled antigen binds only if specific antibody is present to bridge it to the solid phase.

Immunoradiometric Assay (IRMA) is a test for antigen in which excess specific labelled antibody is added to the test antigen. The test antigen binds and neutralizes some of the antibody – the remaining free antibody is removed by adding solid phase antigen. The labelled antibody still in solution is the proportion bound to the test antigen, and the radioactivity of the solution is proportional to the amount of test antigen.

Farr assay uses radiolabelled antigens to detect specific antibody. The test antibody is first mixed with the labelled antigen, then the antibodies are precipitated either using a specific precipitating reagent such as staphylococci which have protein A in their cell walls, or by physicochemical precipitation with ammonium sulphate or polyethylene glycol. The amount of precipitated antigen is proportional to the amount of specific antibody. Some Farr assays use anti-Fc antibodies to precipitate the test antibody. These can be class or subclass specific to detect the amount of specific antibody of a particular isotype.

Enzyme Linked Immunosorbent Assay (ELISA) is used for detecting antibody. Antigen is absorbed to a solid phase and test antibody is added as in the radioimmunoassay, but the ELISA ligand used to detect the antibody is an enzyme linked to a molecule specific for the bound antibody. Enzymes such as peroxidase and phosphatase are often used. In the final stage a chromogenic substrate is added, which generates a coloured end-product in the presence of the enzyme portion of the ligand. The optical density of this solution is measured after a defined period. This is proportional to the amount of the enzyme, which in turn is related to the amount of test antibody. By comparison with RIA, this test has the advantage of stable reagents, but is usually less sensitive.

Homogenous Enzyme Immunoassays (EMIT) are a group of assays to detect antigen using the antigen coupled to an enzyme in such a way that the activity of the enzyme is altered when the antigen binds to the antibody. The antigen/enzyme ligand then competes with the free (test) antigen for a binding site on a limiting

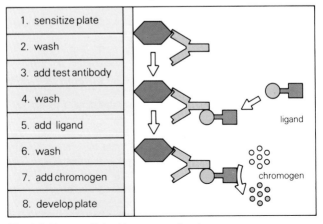

| 1. sensitize plate |
| 2. wash |
| 3. add test antibody |
| 4. wash |
| 5. add ligand |
| 6. wash |
| 7. add chromogen |
| 8. develop plate |

Fig. 6.3 Enzyme linked immunosorbent assay.

amount of antibody, which is also present in the assay mixture (cf. competition radioimmunoassay). In this test it is not necessary to separate bound and unbound antigen.

Fluorescence Immunoassays (FIA) are analagous to radioim-munoassays, but substitute fluoresceinated reagents for the radiola-belled material. The method has the advantage that fluorescent reagents may be detected instantaneously, but problems can arise with the intrinsic fluorescence of the test material and also with the availability of suitable reagents. Some fluorescent reagents respond differently when they are bound to antibody than when free. In this case it is not necessary to separate bound and free fractions of the fluorescent reagent. Examples of this principle include:

Fluorescence quenching is the reduction of fluorescence emit-ted by an antibody (or antigen) when it forms a complex. For example, this occurs when a hapten, which absorbs radiation at 350nm, binds to an antibody. Normally, antibody illuminated at 280nm fluoresces at 350nm, but if the hapten is bound at the bind-ing site some of the fluorescence is absorbed (quenched).

Fluorescence enhancement is the increased fluorescence pro-duced by some haptens when bound to antibody. The energy is absorbed from the antibody and emitted with the wavelength characteristic of the hapten.

Fluorescence polarization. If polarized light is directed at a fluo-rescent molecule it is absorbed and emitted shortly afterwards, during which time the molecules move at random so that the fluorescent emission shows reduced polarization. If, however, the fluorescent molecule is bound to an antibody it has less rotational freedom and the polarization of the emission will be retained to a greater degree.

These properties of fluorescent reagents are used in the determi-nation of antibody affinity and avidity. The determination of anti-body affinity requires that the antigen and antibody react and reach a state of equilibrium. Since it is possible to determine the concen-trations of bound and free fluorescent reagents without separating them, this is a great advantage as physical separation of the free and bound antigen may disturb the equilibrium conditions. Unfortunately suitable fluorescent reagents are available only for a few antigens and antibodies.

Equilibrium dialysis is a method for determining antibody affinity, in which a dialysable antigen or hapten and the test antibody are placed

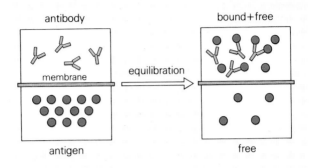

Fig. 6.4 Equilibrium dialysis.

in chambers on opposite sides of a membrane. The system is left until the concentration of free antigen is the same on either side of the membrane (equilibrium), and then the solutions are sampled. The average affinity (K_0) is defined as the reciprocal of the free antigen concentration when half of the antibody's combining sites are occupied; so for IgG with two sites: Affinity, $K_0 = 1/[Ag_{free}]$.

Scatchard equation is the general form for determining antibody affinity: $r/[Ag_{free}] = nK - rK$ where r is the number of antibody sites occupied (i.e. the concentration of bound antigen), n is the antibody valency and K is the affinity constant. Plotting $r/[Ag_{free}]$ against r yields a curve of slope -K which intercepts the r axis at the point where all the antibody combining sites are occupied, that is n, the antibody valency.

Langmuir equation ($1/r = 1/nK. \; 1/[Ag_{free}] + 1/n$) is another formula which can be used to derive the affinity (K_0) and the number of available antibody binding sites (n), by plotting 1/r against $1/[Ag_{free}]$.

Sips equation (log $r/(n-r)$ + a log$[Ag_{free}]$ + a log K_0) can be used to determine affinity (K_0) and the heterogeneity of a population of antibody molecules. Plotting log $r/(n-r)$ against log$[Ag_{free}]$ yields a line with slope = a, which is a measure of the heterogeneity of binding affinity.

Chaotropic dissociation assay is used to measure the heterogeneity of antibody affinities in, for example, serum. Immune complexes are dissociated in buffers of varying strengths at high or low pH or in chaotropic reagents. Low affinity antibodies dissociate in lower strength reagents.

Haemagglutination. This term covers a number of techniques for detecting antibodies, based on the agglutination of red blood cells. The antigen may either be a red cell antigen, or the antigen (sensitizing antigen) required can be chemically linked to the cell surface. For the test, the antibody is titrated in wells and the red cells added. If antibody to the red cell is present the cells are agglutinated and sink as a mat to the bottom of the well, but if it is absent they roll down the sloping sides of the well to form a pellet.

Direct and Indirect Coombs test are the original haemagglutination tests to detect antibodies to red cell antigens, The *direct* Coombs test identifies antibodies which are themselves capable of crosslinking the red cells. The *indirect* Coombs test detects antibodies which cannot crosslink the cells alone (e.g. because there are too few antigens). This is achieved by the addition of a second layer anti-antibody.

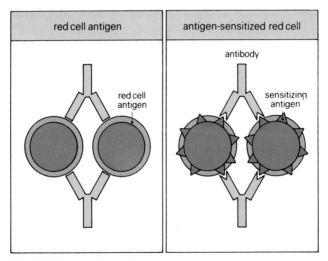

Fig. 6.5 Haemagglutination test.

Complement fixation test detects antibody (or antigen). Test antibody is mixed with the antigen and a small amount of active complement. If antibody is present complexes form and fix the complement, but if none is present active complement remains. Active complement is detected (if complexes did not form) by adding antibody sensitized red cells (EA), which lyse if complement is present. (To detect antigen, specific antibody is mixed with the test solution and complement.)

116

Precipitin reactions. When antigen and antibody react together near their equivalence point they often form crosslinked precipitates. If the reaction occurs in a supporting medium, such as an agar gel, the reactants form precipitin arcs, which can be used to identify antigens and antibodies in complex mixtures.

Immunodouble diffusion (Ouchterlony) is used to distinguish antigens in mixtures. The reactants are placed in holes punched in the gel, and diffuse together. The precipitin arcs may show one of three patterns. Where two arcs are fused this indicates identity between the antigens. If they form independently the antigens are not identical, and if the arcs are fused but with a spur, then the antigens are partially identical, but one antigen contains epitopes which the other lacks.

Countercurrent electrophoresis is a technique for detecting antigens or antibodies by forcing them to move together in an electric field. The technique is related to, but more sensitive than immunodouble diffusion.

Single Radial Immunodiffusion (SRID) (Mancini) is used to quantitate antibody. Test antibody is put in wells in an antigen-containing gel, and diffuses out to form precipitin rings when it reaches equivalence. The area of the ring is proportional to antibody concentration. Antigen can be measured similarly using antibody-containing gels.

Rocket electrophoresis is a modification of SRID in which antigens are quantitated by electrophoresing them through an antibody-containing gel, the pH of which is selected so that the antibodies are neutrally charged and immobile. The antigen moves towards the anode, forming a rocket shaped precipitin arc, where the height of the rocket is proportional to antigen concentrations.

Immunoelectrophoresis (IEP) is a technique in which mixtures of antigen are first separated in an electric field according to their charge, and are then precipitated with anti-serum from a trough lying parallel to the separated antigens.

Crossed electrophoresis (Laurell) first separates antigens according to their charge in an electric field, in the first dimension. Then the antigens are electrophoresed into an antibody-containing gel at right angles to the first separation. In this case the area under the precipitin arcs is proportional to antigen concentration. This technique is useful for quantitating the different forms of an antigen, for example C3 and C3c, which share epitopes but have different charges.

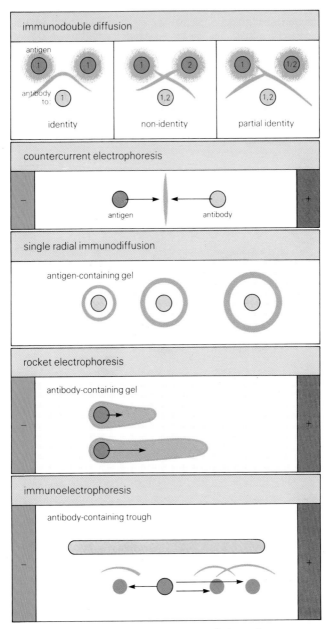

Fig. 6.6 Agar gel immunoprecipitation techniques for identifying antigens and antibody.

Immunoabsorption is used to specifically remove particular antibodies from a solution, by the addition of a solid phase antigen immunoabsorbent.

Immunoabsorbents, that is, solid phase antigens or antibodies, include cells, chemically crosslinked antigen precipitates and proteins coupled to solid supports.

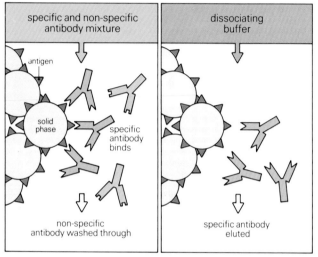

Fig. 6.7 Affinity chromatography.

Affinity chromatography is used to isolate pure antibodies. A column is prepared from antigen covalently coupled to an inert solid phase such as crosslinked dextran beads. The antibody containing solution is run into the column in neutral buffer. Specific antibody binds to the antigen, while unbound antibody and other proteins are washed through. The specific antibody is eluted using a buffer which dissociates the antigen/antibody bond, that is, high or low pH or denaturing agents. By using antibody bound to the solid phase the technique can be used to isolate antigen.

Affinity labelling is used to identify the amino acid residues in an antibody paratope, by the use of special haptens. These haptens have a highly reactive bond which is activated by illumination with UV light. When bound to the antibody these bonds attach to the nearest amino acids, that is, those forming the paratope. The antibody is then denatured and the location of the covalently coupled hapten determined.

Immunofluorescence is a general method for identifying antigens in tissue sections and on cells, or for identifying antibodies to them, as follows:

Direct immunofluoresence. The antibody is covalently coupled to a fluorescent molecule, such as fluorescein or rhodamine, which is then incubated with the cells or a frozen tissue section. The antibody binds to the antigen and this is then visualized by observing the material under a microscope with incident UV light.

Indirect immunofluoresence. In this technique the section is incubated with the test antibody, which is then visualized by the addition of a second layer fluorescent anti-antibody. The amplication produced by the second antibody increases the sensitivity of the assay, and by using class or subclass specific reagents particular isotypes can be identified in the test antibody. This technique is particular valuable for identifying antibodies to tissue antigens, as illustrated below, where antibodies to a pancreatic islet of Langerhans in diabetic serum were identified by indirect immunofluoresence using a frozen section of pancreas.

Capping occurs when antibodies bind and crosslink the surface antigens on a live cell. The antigens aggregate at one pole of the cell, appearing as a (fluorescent) cap. The cap is then internalized (capped off). Treatment of cells with metabolic inhibitors (e.g. azide) prevents capping.

Co-capping is used to determine whether two different cell surface antigens are independent, in which case they form separate caps, with specific antibodies, or associated, when they form a single cap (co-cap).

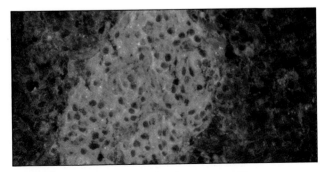

Fig. 6.8 Islet cell autoantibodies demonstrated by immunofluorescence.

ISOLATION OF CELLS

Ficoll gradients are used to isolate cells of different densities. In particular they are used in the purification of lymphocytes. A diluted blood sample is layered onto the Ficoll and centrifuged. Since red blood cells and polymorphs are denser than Ficoll they sediment to the bottom, whilst the lymphocytes and some macrophages remain at the interface. Lymphocyte populations may be further depleted of macrophages by adherence, or by letting the phagocytes take up iron filings and then removing them with a magnet.

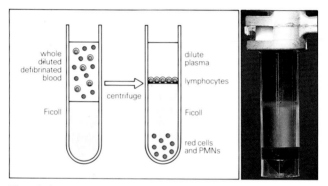

Fig. 6.9 Separation of lymphocytes on a Ficoll isopaque gradient.

Adherence. Macrophages have the property of adhering to plastic, they may be removed from the cell suspensions by plating on plastic dishes to which they adhere.

Panning uses plastic plates sensitized with antigen or antibody (cf. radioimmunoassay). Mixtures of cells are incubated on the plate and cells with receptors for the sensitizing agent bind to it. For example, cells with an antigen receptor will bind to an antigen-coated plate. The technique is often used to deplete cells of a specific subpopulation, but the bound cells can sometimes be recovered by chilling or digesting the plate with enzyme.

Nylon wool adherence is used to fractionate mouse lymphocytes. In physiological conditions, B cells and macrophages adhere to the nylon wool, whereas most T cells do not (some T cell blasts may also adhere). The B cells may be dissociated from the nylon wool by chilling and removing serum from the culture medium.

Rosetting is a method of isolating cells by allowing them to associate with red blood cells. Lymphocytes become surrounded (rosette) with the red cells and may then be isolated by sedimentation through Ficoll gradients.

E Rosettes. Human T cells have receptors for sheep erythrocytes (E) and so may be isolated by mixing with the sheep cells and separating the rosettes produced.

EA Rosettes. Cells which have Fc receptors for IgM or IgG can be isolated by mixing with red cells sensitized with antibody (EA) of the appropriate class. The antibody crosslinks the red cell to the Fc receptor and the rosettes are then isolated.

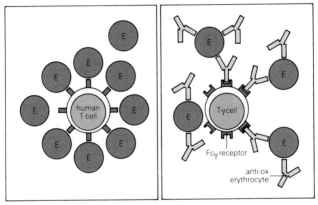

Fig. 6.10 Isolation of cells by rosetting.

Antigen suicide is used to deplete those cells of a population which bind a particular antigen, by supplying them with highly radioactive antigen. This is taken up and kills the cell. A modification of this technique, to kill proliferating cells, is to add bromodeoxyuridine, which they incorporate. Illumination with UV light activates this metabolite to kill the cells.

Antibody/complement depletion. Particular cell populations can be lysed by treatment with specific antibody and complement, activated via the classical pathway.

Fluorescence Activated Cell Sorter (FACS) is a machine which can analyse the size and fluorescence intensity of single cells stained with specific fluorescence antibodies. The cells are then sorted according to these parameters with the exact conditions determined by the operator.

CLONES AND CELL LINES

Clone is a group of cells derived from a single original cell; they are therefore genetically identical.

Line is a group of cells grown in defined conditions from an initially heterogeneous population. Only occasionally will such a line be monoclonal.

Hybridomas are cells produced by the physical fusion of two different cells. Polyethylene glycol and Sendai virus are often used to effect the fusion. A hybridoma cell and its progeny contain some chromosomes from each fusion partner, although some others are usually lost.

Immune responses and antibody populations may be described according to the number of responding cells as:

Monoclonal, Oligoclonal, Polyclonal according to whether it is due to one, a few, or many clones.

Monoclonal antibodies are homogenous antibodies produced by a single clone. They are usually made from hybridomas, which are prepared by fusing immunized mouse or rat spleen cells with a non-secretor myeloma using polyethylene glycol (PEG). The fusion mixture is plated out in HAT medium. HAT contains Hypoxanthine, Aminopterin and Thymidine. Aminopterin blocks a metabolic pathway which can be bypassed if hypoxanthine and thymidine are present, but the myeloma cells lack this bypass and consequently die in HAT medium. Spleen cells also die naturally in culture after 1 - 2 weeks, but fused cells survive since they have the immortality of the myeloma *and* the metabolic bypass of the spleen cells. Some of the fused cells secrete antibody, and supernatants are tested in a specific assay. Wells which produce the desired antibody are then cloned. Human B cells can be immortalized by transformation with Epstein Barr virus.

Cloning by limiting dilution is a process in which a cell population is diluted successively and set up in culture so that there are wells containing only one cell. The progeny of this cell are grown on as a clone.

Cloning from soft agar is done by culturing a cell population in soft agar, which prevents the cells from moving. Colonies which develop around a single cell are removed by micromanipulation and cultured.

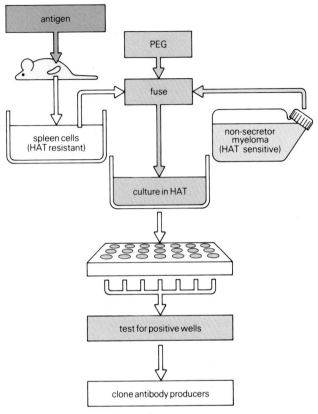

Fig. 6.11 Monoclonal antibody production.

T cell lines are produced by culturing a population of primed T cells in the presence of antigen and/or interleukin-2. The antigen must be presented to the T cells in recognizable form, usually on macrophages which have been treated to block their metabolism. T cell activity is assayed by antigen-specific proliferation.

Proliferation is usually measured by the uptake of radiolabelled metabolites required for DNA or RNA synthesis, such as ^{125}I-uridine deoxyribose or ^{3}H-thymidine. The uptake of these metabolites is measured by harvesting the cells and counting the incorporated radioactivity.

Cell harvester is a machine which semi-automatically aspirates cell cultures, deposits them onto small paper filters and washes away free radioactive metabolites.

CELLULAR FUNCTIONS

Plaque Forming Cells (PFC) are antibody-secreting cells measured in an assay where each secreting cell produces a clear zone of lysis (plaque) in a layer of antigen sensitized red blood cells (see Fig. 6.13).

Indirect plaques measure antigen-specific IgG producers. The test lymphocytes are mixed and incubated with antigen-sensitized red cells (cf. haemagglutination). Antibody from specific B cells binds to the antigen on the red cells, and the addition of antibody to IgG together with complement causes complement fixation on the red cells producing a plaque of lysed cells.

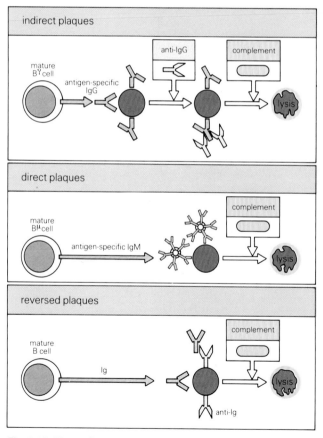

Fig. 6.12 Plaque forming cell assays.

Direct plaques measure the numbers of antigen-specific IgM-producing cells. IgM is capable of fixing complement without the addition of a second layer antibody. Thus IgG and IgM producing cells can be quantitated separately.

Reversed plaques measure the total number of immunoglobulin producing cells (not just the antigen specific ones). Released antibody binds to red cells sensitized with anti-Ig (or protein A). This cell surface complex can now fix complement to produce a plaque.

Elispot assays. These are enzyme immunoassays which are analagous the PFC technique, used to quantitate antigen specific cells. Antibody forming cells are detected by overlaying lymphocytes in agar on a plate sensitized with the specific antigen. Specific antibody binds to the antigen around the cells secreting it. This can then be detected by enzyme immunassay, producing a coloured spot around the active cells. Active T cells can be detected similarly by overlaying them on plates sensitized with antibody to cytokines such as IL-2 or IFN-γ.

Chromium release (cytotoxicity) assay is used to measure the activity of cytotoxic cells. The target cells are first mixed with radioactive ^{51}Cr which is taken up by viable cells. These are then incubated with the test leucocytes. If the test cells damage the targets the ^{51}Cr is released and can be measured in the supernatant.

NBT (Nitroblue Tetrazolium) reduction is a standard test for the oxidative burst in neutrophils.

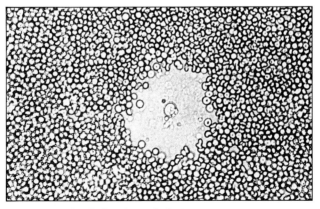

Fig. 6.13 Antibody forming cell plaque.

OTHER COMMONLY USED TECHNIQUES

Immunologists use many biochemical techniques. Some of those more commonly used are outlined below.

Gel filtration/permeation chromatography separates molecules on the basis of size by passing them through columns of microporous beads. Large molecules are excluded from the gel matrix and are eluted first.

Sucrose density gradient ultracentrifugation separates molecules on the basis of their size shape and density.

$CsCl_2$ gradient ultracentrifugation sediments molecules to a point where their density equals that of the $CsCl_2$ gradient, thus separating them on the basis of their buoyant density.

Ion exchange chromatography separates molecules on the basis of their charge. Charged molecules become absorbed to the ion exchange medium and are successively eluted with increasing ion concentration.

Isoelectric Focussing (IEF) analyses molecules according to their isoelectric point (pl), that is, the pH at which the molecule has an overall zero charge.

Spectrotype refers to the characteristic pattern given by a particular molecule separated by IEF. Even monoclonal antibodies produce several lines of different pl, due to post-synthetic modifications.

SDS PAGE (Sodium Dodecyl Sulphate Polyacrylamide Gel Electrophoresis) is a technique to analyse polypeptides according to their size. Proteins treated with SDS become strongly negatively charged and are then electrophoresed through a polyacrylamide gel which acts as a molecular sieve. Since larger peptides bind more SDS, different peptides have similar charge/size ratios and the rate at which they pass through the gel is dependent solely on their size. Smaller molecules are retarded to a lesser degree and migrate fastest.

O'Farrell two dimensional gel separates proteins in an IEF gel in the first dimension and on an SDS polyacrylamide gel in the second, so as to give both the pl and size of the molecules.

Blotting is the technique of transferring proteins separated in polyacrylamide gels onto a reactive 'paper' (e.g. nitrocellulose). Blotted proteins are more readily identified by immunochemical techniques than in the original gels.

Immunoblotting is used to identify blotted proteins by incubating the blot with radiolabelled antibody (or antigen). The antibody binds to antigens on the blot whose location is detected by autoradiography. The bound antibody can also be detected by using a second layer radiolabelled anti-antibody, or enzyme conjugated antibody (cf. radioimmunoassay and ELISA).

Immunoprecipitation is used for characterizing the antigen recognized by a monoclonal antibody, particularly where the antigen is denatured by immunoblotting. The antigen mixture is labelled (radiolabel, biotinylation etc.) and precipitated in solution with the monoclonal antibody and co-precipitating agent (protein A, anti-Ig antibody etc.). The precipitate is then separated on SDS PAGE and the labelled antigen localized.

Autoradiography is used to located radiolabelled materials present in gels or blots, where the test material is directly overlaid with a sheet of film.

Nephelometry is an assay used to detect antigen or antibody by the formation of immune complexes. The complexes make the solution turbid and this can be detected by light scatter.

***In situ* hybridization** is a useful molecular biological technique to detect expression of particular proteins in tissues (e.g. cytokines). Tissue sections are hybridized with radiolabelled cDNA of the protein in question, and the cellular localization of mRNA for that protein determined by autoradiography.

Polymerase Chain Reaction (PCR) is used to amplify small quantities of DNA, by repeated cycles of polymerization. It is useful for generating sufficient DNA for, for example, hybridization or gene cloning, when only small quantities of tissue are available, or when the gene is present in very low quantities.